M000285163

Praise for
Joy Is My Justice

"Dr. Sethi dives into the science behind Joy and reveals the underexplored relationship between mind-body medicine, biochemistry, and Joy. She invites you to learn how to find your power at your very center—and I cannot recommend enough that you accept the invitation."

—Ellen Vora, MD, board-certified holistic psychiatrist and author of *The Anatomy of Anxiety*

"Let this be your most transformative journey of healing yet—one that starts from the inside out. Dr. Sethi's road map to Joy is the most sacred medicine you will find. She beautifully shows us how ancient wisdom can be amplified through the lens of Justice to create a guide for not only surviving your pain, but for thriving through Joy."

—Avanti Kumar-Singh, MD, Ayurvedic physician and author of *The Healing Catalyst*

"*Joy Is My Justice* is a clear-eyed, eloquent, loving guide to the Joy and fulfillment that we can discover as we meet life's darkest, most traumatizing challenges. Tanmeet Sethi has been there and done that. She does it every day, and generously shares her hard-earned wisdom."

—James S. Gordon, MD, author of *Transforming Trauma: The Path to Hope and Healing and Founder* and CEO of The Center for Mind-Body Medicine

"If you have ever struggled with life's challenges (and who hasn't?); if your inner critic regularly berates you (and whose doesn't?) this is the book for you. Heartbreaking and triumphant, *Joy Is My Justice* maps a courageous and compassionate path forward with practices we can all learn and do."

—Victoria Maizes, MD, executive director, Andrew Weil Center for Integrative Medicine, University of Arizona, author of *Be Fruitful: The Essential Guide to Maximizing Fertility and Giving Birth to a Healthy Child*

Joy Is My Justice

Joy Is My Justice

RECLAIM WHAT IS YOURS

TANMEET SETHI, MD

NEW YORK

Note: The information in this book is true and complete to the best of our knowledge. This book is intended only as an informative guide for those wishing to know more about health issues. In no way is this book intended to replace, countermand, or conflict with the advice given to you by your own physician. The ultimate decision concerning care should be made between you and your doctor. We strongly recommend you follow their advice. Information in this book is general and is offered with no guarantees on the part of the authors or Hachette Go. The authors and publisher disclaim all liability in connection with the use of this book.

Cover design by Terri Sirma

Hachette Go, an imprint of Hachette Books
Hachette Book Group
1290 Avenue of the Americas
New York, NY 10104
HachetteGo.com
Facebook.com/HachetteGo
Instagram.com/HachetteGo

First Edition: May 2023

Hachette Books is a division of Hachette Book Group, Inc.

The Hachette Go and Hachette Books name and logos are trademarks of Hachette Book Group, Inc.

The Hachette Speakers Bureau provides a wide range of authors for speaking events.

To find out more, go to hachettespeakersbureau.com or email HachetteSpeakers@hbgusa.com.

Hachette Go books may be purchased in bulk for business, educational, or promotional use. For information, please contact your local bookseller or Hachette Book Group Special Markets Department at special.markets@hbgusa.com.

The publisher is not responsible for websites (or their content) that are not owned by the publisher.

Library of Congress Cataloging-in-Publication Data has been applied for.

ISBNs: 978-0-306-83003-7 (hardcover); 978-0-306-83005-1 (ebook)

LCCN: 2022051038

Printed in the United States of America

LSC-C

Printing 1, 2023

For my deepest river of love—Neha, Zubin, Sahaj, and Steve

Contents

Author's Note

Before we begin, I'd like to acknowledge two things:

- Some names have been changed for privacy; some patient stories are composites.
- The practices you'll find throughout these pages are not fully of my or any contemporary teacher's creation; they are fundamentally rooted in global traditions and lineages (inclusive of Indigenous Americas, Africa, Asia, and the South Pacific) and amplified here with loving reciprocity.

Prologue

I was nine months pregnant with my third child, on top of the world, when my dreams suddenly shattered. My barely three-year-old son, Zubin, was handed a death sentence: Duchenne muscular dystrophy... like an ALS in children. In a moment that can never be undone, my life was time-stamped into a *before* and an *after*.

Everyone alive will endure great pain—multiple times and usually beyond our control. What we choose to do with that pain is critical. Escape was my first impulse. Running away is our most primal survival tactic. But I learned that, if instead I choose to walk back toward my pain, something radical, even revolutionary, could emerge: Joy.

That work of finding and keeping Joy, no matter what, has become my most potent medicine. A medicine that is accessible to all, independent of race, gender expression, or bank account. Joy is your birthright... even when your child is dying, right before your eyes.

As a Sikh American physician and activist, I have spent the last two and a half decades working in the most underserved communities, fighting for health equity through racial, gender, and food justice. I seek Justice through the medical, legal, or social outcome of my efforts. But in this book, the battleground for

Justice is *our own lives, our own bodies*, where we can find Joy no matter what our external circumstances are.

Your pain is not fair or just. You are not broken because you feel it deeply. Yet every footstep you take toward Joy, even while still living with fear or rage, is a radical act of Justice that defies the oppressive weight of your pain and creates a powerful change in your biochemistry. You and only you choose which neurochemical will take strongest hold in your brain and heart; you choose what story your cells will hear.

I do not mean that you should accept inequity or injustice as unchangeable truths. Just the opposite. When you find your own Joy and create a personal path for Justice—which only you can forge—you are better able to right unfairness in the world because you have risen into your own power first. You move from contraction to openness, from someone who was held back to one who moves forward. My determination to find Joy has healed other deep wounds in my life—despite my grief and cultural guilt that a mother should not be Joyful if her child is dying. Joy is that powerful a medicine. *Joy is my Justice.*

When your personal Justice begins in your body, you are in liberation work daily. You see clearly a broken world of wellness and self-empowerment that is predicated on an oppressive ideology: if you do not feel good, it is because you are not *good enough* at getting better. This world is unjust. Systems are often built against you. And bad things happen, to all of us.

And yes, this Justice work is hard. I won't lie. When you repave old patterns, your body can be confused and uncomfortable; like laying down new roads, it's tiring and sweaty work. But receive this: This kind of feeling bad is a signal you want, it signifies a new beginning, a new path you are paving. Get familiar with this feeling, be it a signal of discomfort, anxiety, or fear. It is a message from your body that it hears your call for a new way. It's time to let your pain be the alchemy for the life you were meant to live.

You can learn to linger in Joy so that your body and entire intricate nervous system bathe in its magic and remember it more easily in times of struggle. Not because your struggle isn't real (*It always is*), not because you ever need to dampen any difficult emotions (*Those are also real and vital*), but instead because having Joy as your steady companion expands your capacity to hold it all.

This is the book I wish I'd had to read as a young Brown girl who internalized hate from the world around me. And later in life on a mother's nightmarish day, to give me hope and faith that my family's life was not over. And this is the story the world desperately needs right now: Joy is here if you want a relationship with her. But she's not going to just knock on your door. You have to find a way to open to her. And when you do, you reclaim Joy in your own body, where Justice has always lived.

Joy is here for *you*.

Joy is your birthright.

It's my mission to make sure you find *yours*.

And this book will lead you there.

That Monday

It started out like any Monday. Monday, September 24, 2007, to be exact. That afternoon, I walked into my colleague's office with a frozen look and told him in a monotone voice to cancel my patients that afternoon.

I have to leave... now.

Those were the only words I could find. Steve, my husband, had just called, with only three words for me.

Come home... now.

His voice quivered slightly, and it was the quiver that left me frozen.

Steve holds an unwavering faith in life. It's sometimes quite annoying to my anxiety and doom-prone self, but it serves him, and our family, well. As an anesthesiologist, he's the calm in the storm. Every time my children and I are at a work gathering, someone will tell us that Steve is *the guy we want in the operating room when things are going wrong.* We make bets on how many times we'll be asked, *Does he* ever *get mad?* He's that guy whose heart may be racing on the inside, but on the outside, he looks placid, unshakable.

So, when Steve trembles, you know things have already gone very wrong.

Just a week earlier, Zubin's physical therapist had confronted me at his developmental preschool. *Something more is going on* is what she said. I felt her five words suffocating me. As if she had reached straight into my heart and painfully nudged my deepest fear.

Something is going on, I had said so many times to Steve over those last two and a half years of Zubin's life. And of course, he would pacify me with his reassurances and faith in the good.

I think he's fine. (Okay, if Steve isn't worried, I feel reassured.)

All children develop at their own pace. You take care of young children, you know that. (Yes, using my medical expertise as a distraction worked many times.)

We can't compare him to Sahaj. (And of course, the most effective one, calling the comparison card.)

Our precocious older son, Sahaj, not only reached every milestone early, but he was already saying things wise beyond his years. His brother, Zubin, had yet to run, had taken a long time to even walk, and was still speaking only a few words. Yet I would sigh with relief when Steve would allay my worries. It was as if his ease gave me permission to discard any scary premonitions I had. *If Steve is calm, all must be okay.*

And so it came to pass that my husband called on that Monday with a wavering in his voice that I had never heard before.

Come home now.

Steve waited for me on our front porch on that warm fall day. It was as if he didn't want to utter the words inside our home. We didn't make it past the wooden glider bench, given to us by close friends when we finally became parents. *When you were born, our hearts rejoiced*, the engraving proclaimed, implying Joy was surely to follow.

In one prick of a needle, one blood test had shattered everything that bench had promised, every milestone, every anticipated marvel of this journey of parenting. No, this would not be how we had imagined it.

Muscular dystrophy.

Duchenne muscular dystrophy (DMD).

Those were the three words we were now left with. Of all the eighty-plus types, it was the most severe, the fatal one, the kind that would deteriorate and ravage Zubin's body.

DMD is a mutation in the longest gene in the human body, dystrophin, the main building block for all muscle. Leg, arm, lung, heart. All of it. Boys with DMD lose their ability to walk until eventually their lungs and heart fail. It is a disease that no mother, including a doctor mother, wants to read about or comprehend.

On an otherwise sunny September Monday, one month before the birth of our third child no less, my life got way less perfect. Permanently less perfect.

And nobody's clichéd sympathies, homemade casseroles, or positive thinking would bring me any closer to jumping over this kind of hurdle.

A Road Map

I recently had a vision, I mean the *this-can't-be-real-someone-must-be-messing-with-me* kind. No, I don't usually have visions. I've led at least a thousand people in a practice to meet their inner, wise guides and I swear, even people who have never meditated in their life come out of that with images of sacred owls and all kinds of amazing messages, grandmothers in light form, the whole bit. And me? Nothing. How I came to this particular vision is a longer story for another time, but I was cradled in a lush golden sling, at least that's the best I can describe it, my head held by my *masi* (Mom's sister) who is no longer on this earth, and my feet by my son, Zubin, who lives, but tenuously. They were lovingly rocking me over an abyss that symbolized the unknown (you just know that kind of shit in a vision) and saying, almost chanting, to trust and then trust some more. To trust the rattling uncertainty in my life, to know that a path would unfold, and that I could be bold enough to follow it.

This book is a threshold over your own abyss, over that liminal space between *what is no longer for you* and *what is yet to be.* Helluva scary place to dangle, but you can knit your own wide, golden sling. The truth is, you walk through these transitions all the time—between jobs, after scary diagnoses, relationships shattered or discovered, unspeakable events, through all the befores and afters—into the unfolding of your life. This time, walk with me into the unknown and trust that Joy is not only yours to have but that a Joy discovered through the lens of Justice may be the most enduring you can find.

Yes, we will lay out the practice of Joy. But not the usual whitewashed, oversimplified one of a wellness patriarchy that ignores the oppressive world and deems that Joy is for the most *resilient*, for the human beings who are able to rewire their brain and shift their thoughts. First of all, that requires privilege—nothing wrong with that, but let's call it out. You can't positively think your way out of poverty, dangerous situations, or oppression. Second, Joy already lives and flows in your body where rational cognition does not govern. Just as your body does not need your willful thought to exert its most primal functions, so does Joy not need to be given to you by someone else. Third and possibly most important, none of us has asked for suffering. Suffering isn't a personal or moral failing or the result of a faulty nervous system. We are merely humans who have experienced tragedy brought on by other humans, natural disasters, failed systems, or sheer fate, and it is *these tragedies* that have oppressed and dysregulated our nervous system. We've experienced a lack of safety; our mind, heart, and body have done—and continue to do—what they lovingly needed to get us through it.

Time-out for a medical disclaimer: I'm a physician who has tended to countless humans in deep suffering and has seen the depths of challenge it can take to even care about trying to survive. I'm also a human who has suffered from clinical depression, more than once. I know what it's like to lie in bed and wonder why the hell even bother to get up. One of my bouts almost ruined two other lives in the process.

This book is not a comprehensive treatment for depression, complex trauma, or post-traumatic stress disorder (PTSD). It is not a substitute for medications or supplements, trauma-informed counseling, or work with a somatic therapist. If you're using those, use them well and lovingly. They can be lifesavers. Honor and have gratitude for them, but even with the grace of those offerings, know that there are still more tools available to you.

This is about you taking Justice into your own hands, into your own body. This is about finding your path to Joy, not through platitudes or contrived positivity, but instead through settling more peacefully in your skin. That is revolutionary Justice: finding your own sense of safety when the world has denied it to you. And if we want more Justice in the world at large, we all need to feel more of this liberation in our body first. So, let's reclaim some important language.

JOY

The Joy we will speak of is not only about feeling better than you do today, but instead about feeling more…

More Power, not of the colonial hierarchal sort, but of the personal, revolutionary kind.

More Connection, not only to others, but to yourself, where the most power resides.

More Belonging, to something greater than whatever gave rise to your pain in the first place.

This Joy is not the same as happiness.

Happiness is a cognitive construct, an evaluation of how life is going. Joy is not intellectual. It draws on the same deep well as your pain, on your capacity for love and meaning. Joy is what your body knows and has always known.

This Joy is not about getting somewhere.

Or wishing things were different. Or even getting rid of the hard things. It is not a solution. It's a way to hold all the questions.

This Joy is not a commodity that you seek in a luxurious spa.

It is not a service that you must make more time and money for. Joy lives inside you and expands the time you already have.

This Joy is a touchstone that you can come back to over and over, an infinite inner resource.

You don't have to be Joyful all the time. I sure as hell am not. You just need to know how to access Joy repeatedly. When you stray from it, it is not a failure. It's an invitation to stray back and touch it again, like a soothing mantra. Joy grounds you in something bigger than all the challenging emotions; it's what you need to live this beautiful and horrible life.

This Joy is not binary.

When you're experiencing the pain of loss, grief, injustice, or oppression, you deserve moments (and even longer) of Joy, Hope, and Love at the same time. The greater your pain, the more necessary it is for you to find your way to them. And here's the real truth: When you lovingly meet pain in your body, you will reclaim your power. Your life struggles may not have been ones you chose, but you can use your lived pain to *your advantage* now.

This Joy does not negate the potent truth of your anger, fear, or grief.

These emotions are necessary protectors and messengers to make change in your life, and then in the world. No forced positivity here. Just the opposite: open to that pain, yours and the world's alike, so that you can feel the Joy more deeply. And then let your Joy practice create an island of Justice in your body first, where it matters the most. This Joy does not crowd out or do away with your pain. Instead, it creates space so your hold on it is less tense.

You do not have to "earn" this Joy.

Don't let that old and tired lie live on. Joy is a fundamental human right that you are *entitled* to, the most primal Justice you will ever know. And now is the time to seize it.

This Joy also does not come only when all else in the world is right.

Every step to Joy is a sweet gift of long-overdue equity, the payback we all deserve *right now*. Each time you connect to the universal energy of Joy, you create a deeper sense of belonging in and connection to this world that you have every right to inhabit. Joy is your defiant battle cry. I wish I had known so long ago that finding safety in my own body would pave the way for fighting for it on all other territory.

I write this book into 2022, in the ongoing COVID-19 pandemic and continued racial injustice, the overturning of *Roe v. Wade*, and the possibility of shattering who knows what other civil rights after that. There are kinds of pain that may make an invitation to Joy downright hurtful and offensive. Hear me with love: Joy is not about creating a false reality. It's about finding something within you even greater and more meaningful than that injustice, that then you can toll as the loudest bell in your body until you recognize that your own Joy was hidden underneath the entire time.

JUSTICE

What does Justice mean to you? What would it feel like to receive it? Take a moment to reflect on that.

In these pages, I invite you to a fight for your Justice that gives grace for every ounce of pain you have endured, every time you have been asked to be resilient yet again, and also every step you take toward Joy alongside all that.

If the painful truths of your life are unchangeable, as many are, I feel you deeply. Joy is still, and even more, critical because no healing can start in your body without the soothing, cleansing energy of knowing you are so much more than your tragedies and difficult stories. Joy is an act of *resistance*, your own internal revolution, which then allows you to right unfairness in the world. Searching for fairness will decimate your spirit but seeking the Justice of Joy will save your soul.

If you are someone who has been pushed to the margins of or excluded in conversations on health and wellness, this book centers your experience and is a love letter to you. As a Sikh, Desi woman, I carry both the deep oppression of my colonized past as well as a complex history of internalized alignment with whiteness. With the privilege of writing this book, I stand on the shoulders of all my Black, Brown, and Indigenous ancestors, amplifying ancient wisdom with sincere reciprocity. This is not a book on racism but being a Brown woman means that race shows up in all that I am and all that I heal.

If you carry white or other privilege, you're also welcomed lovingly to learn, do your own work, and then wield your power wisely. Your liberation has always been intricately tied to all others. You, like me, may carry inherited or acquired power. In this journey, I invite you to join me in leaving guilt or shame at the door; they won't serve you here.

LIBERATION

When I speak of liberation, I don't mean the clichéd promise of a red-white-and-blue-washed American freedom. I mean the capacity to face your pain, hold it gently, and then use it as rocket fuel for your personal revolution: to feel Joy, love yourself, embrace hope, and know you deserve all this and more.

I've worked with countless humans, some whom you will meet in this book, who have endured countless traumas, and again and again, they prove we all have the capacity for a more Joyful life. We *all* deserve Joy, no matter where we sit or how we suffer, and the world needs yours. Let your revolution ignite all others.

I want you to feel liberation even as you travel the liminal space of these pages. To read as slowly or quickly as you choose, to skip around as you feel called. There are breaks to *Take a Pause* offered along the way as space for reflection on the concepts; this is your journey to forge. Rest is crucial. If you can, take a moment and breathe into the pauses, letting them sink into your body. At the end of sections, when relevant, there are offerings of *Practices*. No requirements or pressure, take any or none. I describe those exercises in writing so you can read and then do them as feels right to you. When relevant, I also offer them in guided audio format on my website (www.tanmeetsethimd.com) if you choose to listen to me walk you through them. This book is a guide to *your* Joy. That means you have the right to find it how you like.

Let's take a tour of the road map ahead.

Part 1 is an opportunity to reflect on what may be blocking Joy in your life, what is no longer for you, and what you can embrace instead. Removing barriers and creating room for healing is always the first step so you can then take up the space you were always entitled to. Take deep breaths, and often. As I wrote this book, I sure as hell did.

Part 2 lays out tools to access your Joy, reframed through the lens of your Justice. One or more may be the gateway or window to your unique revolution. If you need more support or safety on this path from trained professionals or loving community, please do seek it from those you trust and who can make space for all you are. This is not a journey to travel alone. The path to Joy often reveals your most profound vulnerabilities. But make no mistake, this exploration of facing discomfort and, at times, unsettling physical sensations, and learning not to be overwhelmed by them, is the magic of how you liberate your body from the tangled pain itself.

Part 3 guides you to reclaim and integrate Joy as a steady life practice. Learning to unapologetically practice Joy feels at times like an unfamiliar balance and at others a freeing of energy deep in your body. The thoughts come up, *I don't deserve this (especially when others are suffering)*, *This feels too hard*, or *Why bother?* Until you find your balance and *know* it instead of overthinking it. When you commit to Joy as a practice in your life, you embody a way of seeing yourself that then changes how you see the world. It moves from your head as an intellectual exercise to your body as known fabric, weaving it in as *utter trust* that you are capable and deserving of Joy each and every day. Your nervous system's most powerful vagus nerve is 80 percent afferent, which is fancy speak for 80 percent of its fibers coming *from the body to the brain* and not the reverse. In fact, the heart and the gut have been described in mainstream medical literature as each literally *having their own brain*. ***What you do in your body rewrites how your brain interprets and translates your life.***

Joy is your birthright, no matter what has been given to you. You can retrieve a knowing that is primal and deep to your core and feels truer than any teaching from outside yourself ever has. Your will to thrive and flourish becomes your core personal revolutionary practice. And if all this sounds *too big* or *too much* to hope for, think on this. All revolutions kindle first in our imagination, in our dreams. Until our body can ignite them with our hope and love. Let yourself imagine what is possible, let yourself dream of too much instead of too little. It's time to take up the *big* space you were always entitled to.

PART I

RECLAIM YOUR SPACE

CHAPTER 1

Does Joy Matter?

WHY F—ING BOTHER?

Maxine was a patient in our clinic, a mild-mannered woman in her late forties but her weathered face and slow gait fooled you to think she had been through more than four decades should give anyone. She joined my mind body medicine group and was skeptical that anything we learned could help ease her decades of chronic back pain. But my colleague, her family physician, had pleaded with her to please try. *Nothing else was working anyway,* she told Maxine. She explained that this group was a place to learn new tools, ones that didn't come in bottles or needles. Pain had become such a part of her life that Maxine admitted in the first group her personal feeling of futility for even being here and wondered out loud if this was a waste of time. The fourth week in, we were doing a writing exercise in which you dialogue with something in your life, a physical, emotional, or spiritual symptom that you are bothered by or wondering about, and ask it questions. It feels like a screenplay of sorts where you keep pen to paper and have the *symptom* talk, even if it feels contrived at first, until you get answers.

Out of everyone in the group, she was the most doubtful about this practice. The skepticism wasn't anything new; this exercise often confused participants. *I don't get it, aren't we just talking to ourselves? This seems crazy.* I assured her it could sound that way, but invited Maxine to open her mind and heart and just try it out. Even if nothing gained, nothing lost in the process, other than fifteen minutes of time with pen to paper. She conceded. After we were done, I asked everyone to reread their writing silently to themselves and see whether they had a message or takeaway. I then invited whoever was interested to read it out loud to us and explained that this could be an even more profound way of processing the exercise.

This was the hardest part, the most vulnerable ask, so I was used to no one jumping out of their seat to accept my invitation. After only a few moments of silence, I was surprised that the first inclination came from Maxine.

I don't want to read my whole thing out loud. But I do want to share something. I started this exercise thinking it was crazy and that never changed through the whole thing.

Her response earned a calming chuckle from the group.

And then the weirdest thing happened. I was writing about how stupid this was and my hand started changing. She stopped talking and looked down.

Do you want to share more about that? I asked.

Well, she went on, still staring at the floor, *what was crazy was that my hand started writing like I was a little girl. Literally my hand started writing like the way I did when I was seven. And I couldn't stop it. I don't want to talk about what I was writing because I didn't like it. I didn't like my life when I was seven. And I still didn't like it now.*

Again, silence, this time a thicker one. Slowly, she raised her head, her eyes wet.

But something even crazier happened when that little girl took over. For the first time in so long that I can't even remember, my pain went away.

You could have heard a pin drop in that room.

It's coming back a little now. But for that time, it all went away. That shit is crazy.

The group relaxed into laughter.

I stayed silent to see whether there was more.

For the first time in so long, I saw that maybe, just maybe, there's a chance for me. Even though the pain is coming back, I just had fifteen minutes of peace and I'm going to take that for now. I've been trying every medicine and doctor, but this is power I didn't know I had.

The entire group in that moment exhaled at the same time as if her epiphany meant maybe, just maybe, we all had that power as well.

You can wax poetic on all kinds of Freudian or other psychology theory of why Maxine's handwriting changed and why her pain went away with it. The theories aside, studies show when you write, not about the logistical or mundane parts of your day, but instead about emotionally troubling life events, big magic can happen. Magic like less depression, stronger immune systems, and even clinical changes in chronic diseases, such as asthma or rheumatoid arthritis. One of the most prolific researchers of this effect, social psychologist James W. Pennebaker, speculated that especially when you write about a long-suppressed secret, the physiological changes may be even more profound.

Suffering makes your world small, narrow, unsolvable. It's hard to see a way out because you can barely look at what's in front of you. But your body has both the desire and the wisdom to heal and reclaim space for more than just the pain that has taken up residence for so long. Maxine was untangling so much underneath that didn't require analysis in that moment, just our presence.

Maxine's sliver of suffering expanded, first for just that fifteen minutes, but it was enough to widen so she could see the possibility for more. That her Justice didn't need to come only from others, that maybe deep within the well of her body, it had lived in her all the time.

Looking for Joy expands your world and when it does, you can see more—more reason to keep seeking until you live your way into a world that feels worth fighting for.

Take a Pause

You deserve the same kind of expansiveness, and the world deserves you expanding into it. If you're in that small sliver of suffering right now, let's work with that and see what can emerge.

You may want to run away from your current unbearable sliver as fast as possible. That's normal. You aren't weak or avoidant. Your heightened nervous system is just vigilant and uncomfortable, and you want to extinguish those sensations through the more comfortable paths of distraction and escape. This is coded into your DNA: *be cautious of danger or pain and avoid it*. It's how our ancestors survived. It's how you protect yourself from hot stoves and shards of glass. If you do brave the journey toward your pain, the science supports that you carve new pathways in your nervous system best by going slow. It is okay to tread lightly.

Especially if you've been in a state of withdrawal, overwhelmed by your life's history and pain, take a deep breath with a long exhale. That sigh signals to your body that you are here to carve new channels that recognize your pain and something radically different, both rooted in the same capacity to love and care. From the alchemy of your pain and power, Joy can emerge. That is the revolution.

When I ask myself on my hardest days if Joy is worth fighting for, a question that still comes up more than I would like, I often reflect on a visit, several years ago, to one of the largest concentration camps in Germany. In the camp's barren and eerie expanse of broken concrete, there was a flower that grew through one endless crack. The contrast of a lone yellow flower to the pure evil that had surrounded it was so stark that my entire family stopped silent to marvel at its baffling will to exist. How did it survive? And why would it even *want* to exist here? We didn't have the answer, but that image remains a symbol to me of what can emerge from the hollow ground of evil. That this flower could be getting enough life force was both a wonder and an inspiration. There is always a reason worth fighting for, whether it's to thrive or to inspire. Whether it's to prove to no one other than yourself that this one life is worth existing for.

WHAT IS YOUR DEEPER WHY?

There's just no room for it, Dr. Sethi, you know that.

Janelle sat across from me in the exam room, a signature green logo to-go cup in one hand and her phone in the other. Coffee had become her constant companion since giving up vices far more damaging. Her phone within reach, in case her mom finally called. She looked down immediately after speaking as if facing me would make the truth even more painful. She was alone today, without her kids, and noticeably more sullen.

I sat, stunned. Not because I was surprised by what she said, but because I felt it so very deeply in my body. A truth resonated through my chest, hollowing out a space inside me. My fear that Janelle was actually right filled the emptiness.

Yes, I knew that she had a very hard life. Poverty, chronic illness, and the ever-looming threat of drug addiction relapse took up any space remaining after caring for her kids, fighting to put food on the table, and managing the unpredictable calls from her mom whose own dangerous addiction remained an ever-present reality. The entire extended family were my patients, so I knew all too well what little space there was.

And yet I had asked.

How can you make space for Joy in your life?

There's just no room for it, Dr. Sethi.

My brothers, to this day, tease me about my childhood love for the movie *Rocky*. I would watch it over and over, suffering through Stallone's grunts and mediocre acting, and *still* cry every time. Even though I knew the ending was the same, every time. It wasn't just *Rocky*. I get teary and "Eye of the Tiger" kind of fired up with any underdog story.

It isn't any surprise I would become a physician who labors for social justice and takes care of the most vulnerable. I'm at my best and most alive when I fight with those in the shadows.

My parents were cautious about my choice of medicine as a career. A bad business decision, they told me, to take out that many loans (they weren't wrong about that). And of course, it would mean I might wait *too* long to get married (that's up for debate). But I insisted. Not because I had a love of science (that was furthest from the truth; I still shudder when I think about organic chemistry). Not because I had any role models (there were no doctors in my entire extended family, not a one). And truth be told, I wasn't even sure I could survive cutting up dead bodies in an anatomy lab. (Even in my one summer spent volunteering in a hospital, I was nauseous every day from the over-sanitized hallways and formaldehyde scents.) Nothing about my decision made logical sense. I went on a hunch. I knew I wanted to do right in this world, serve the underdog, and acquire power to make change. Being a physician felt like the way to get this all done.

By all appearances, you might then think I'm a *good person*. That I help people and do right in this world. That last part is true, I am proud of that. But I advocate for others simply because it helps me.

You see, I have never felt safe in this world. I lived a childhood of not belonging, a timid first-generation Brown Indian girl in the US South, shuttling between a home in which our culture persevered as strongly as in the 1960s India my parents had left and an unknown world that they fiercely protected me from. I felt out of sorts in both. Too American for my Indian community and too Brown for my American circles. Growing up, my brothers and I were harassed constantly in school for *the tennis ball on their head* (referring to their turban) or our *Halloween costumes* (to this day, I fiercely avoid costume parties). I embarrassingly admit I would walk with my family in public enough distance away so they wouldn't worry I was too far, but far enough that maybe, just maybe, passersby wouldn't think I was with them. Racists littered our lives, including ones who gave my father death threats, right in front of us.

Random white man: *Are you from I-ran?*

My father: *No.*

Man: *Good, because I have a gun and was going to kill you if you said yes.*

On days like that, we just walked away... briskly. Those moments and many in between put me in a hypervigilant state, creating a constant gas-pedal push on my stress system. To this day, I look around more than my friends do on a new street corner, watching my back, constantly.

When I was ten, the FBI came to our home one night to investigate whether my father was part of a local financing plot for an assassination attempt of a visiting Indian official. (For the record, the answer is still no.) They questioned two other elders in our community and even went out of their way to tail us for a couple of days. I have such a strong memory of sitting on the steps outside the room they met in, trying to eavesdrop and wondering if they could take my father away. The fear is still palpable in my chest. His innocence didn't matter. We were all terrorists to them.

Our home was broken into multiple times. Even after our getting an alarm system, someone cut through a wooden door panel to get in and not trip the alarm tape on the windows. People in my neighborhood were assaulted and raped. Our friend, a local middle school teacher, carried a gun to school. I suffered from insomnia, unable to guide my nervous system to any ease.

My father would always tell us his plan for our family to return to India where our culture could be lived *intact*. Until 1984, when a genocide played out against our people there. Then, there was no going back. My parents, who lived through the Partition as children and had already fled one land, knew what this meant. Now, here we were to stay, he told us. In a country that didn't truly accept us but with no home to return to either.

I used to at least feel comfortable in our *gurdwaras*, our places of worship. The room where we pray to *Waheguru* (God) and sit and sing from our holy book, the *Guru Granth Sahib*. But on August 5, 2012, that was taken away, too, when a gunman entered the gurdwara in Oak Creek, Wisconsin, and shot Sikhs as they prayed. In the only room that was still sacred. Now, I sit strategically in gurdwaras, where I can see the door.

I am a scared person who has desperately wanted to feel safe in my body. And since I could never do that, I now realize I have tried to make the world right for others, subconsciously hoping this would make it safer for me.

On that Monday, when the world crashed down on me in a way I had never experienced before, I could not imagine finding Joy ever again. Because after Zubin was diagnosed, there was nothing to fight against. No oppressive system that could hopefully change, not a disease that even had a chance at a miracle. DMD was fatal, 100 percent. No cure. No use trying. This was it. Nowhere to run, nowhere to feel safe, and no one to fight for... but myself.

I wish I could go back to that day with Janelle and tell her what I know now. That Joy is not made-up Neverland fairy dust that you sprinkle and, suddenly, life feels okay. Joy is not about finding the *right* outcome or having the *right* mind-set. It's more powerful than that. And it was her right to make space for Joy all the while.

I wish I could go back and guide Janelle to find her own deeper why that made sense to her, why she needed and deserved Joy in her life. When you reveal this deeper layer to yourself, your brain makes the process simpler. When you know this why, your brain comes back and recommits to it more easily when life gets more stressful, which it will. Your brain wants the easiest path always, that's why you run away and avoid. But you can carve a new one with this anchor, so that holding Joy becomes less like work and more like you. Because no matter how much you commit to this path, trust me, at some point, you will wonder, *Why f— bother?*

I wish I could tell Janelle that as deep as my why is to serve in medicine, even deeper now is my mission to share with you how to access Joy. In fact, both have become my Justice work in this world. I don't wait anymore for this life to be fair or just. I seize it as such. But it took me the kind of pain that brings a mother to her knees to realize my lifelong thirst for Joy was misguided. It could not only be dependent on systems changing, on ignorance resolving, or having a *good* life. Instead, I had to find the Joy that there is always room for, the Joy that already lives in my body. Joy waits for the day you finally believe in her because doing so means you believe in yourself.

I'm not a human who seeks Joy only because I have pain.

I seek it because I know that no one else can save me.

PRACTICE: YOUR DEEPER WHY

Finding your own Deeper Why will help you stay committed to this path, especially when life is stressful. Even if the answer feels obvious to you, try this exercise and you may be surprised by what you uncover. I usually am.

1. The basic premise of the practice is to ask yourself, *Why*, over and over. In this case, it may be *Why bother finding Joy* when your life continues to offer pain. *What is the point or purpose? Why is it worth it to me? Why do I deserve to find Joy?* Or you may have a different question you are asking. Write out the question or plant it firmly in your heart.
2. You can do this in a journal, during meditation or prayer states, or even while doing a moving meditation, such as running, walking, biking, or rolling in your wheelchair. If you cannot

write, you can speak it into a voice memo app on your phone. Whatever way works for you.

3. Note the answer each time, take a pause, maybe a breath, and then ask *But, Why* again as a response to that reason.
4. Ask *Why* at least five to seven times, but as many as you need to feel complete. You may even feel this completeness in your body as a chill or goose bumps or as a feeling of expansiveness or lightness.
5. Feel free to post the deepest layer you reach somewhere you can see it often, access it again in a meditative state, or even shred any evidence. This is all for you.

CHAPTER 2

You're Not Broken

THE SYSTEM IS

In my social Justice work, I often say that the systems we are fighting against are not in fact broken; they are unfortunately very good at doing what they have been designed to do.

The systems of your body are also not broken. It's worth taking a deeper dive into this science because it is Justice of its own to understand your body and how it helps you survive any great pain or loss. In the moments or days of the most acute pain, your nervous system works to help you fight, flee, or even freeze into a numb state to withstand the enormity of the event. It's your body's intricate power, a delicate design to flow between states of calm and vigilance in the span of the same day or even hour. Your autonomic nervous system consists of the sympathetic (stress) and parasympathetic (rest and digest) systems. When you react to something as big as the proverbial tiger or as mundane but persistent as the nagging hardships of your daily life, stress hormones spill into your body, revving up your sympathetic system. You need this stimulus to save you from danger but also for daily living, to mobilize you to stay alert and focused.

All parts of your wondrous nervous system are there for good reason. Including the longest nerve of the body, your parasympathetic vagus nerve, named from the Latin word for *wandering*, that travels from the base of your brain stem through your entire face and down to the deepest organs of your gut. Author and trauma expert Resmaa Menakem refers to it as the *soul nerve*. It is the deepest seed of our body, the way we connect to this world and ourselves.

Take a Pause

Let's take a moment to exhale a breath of gratitude for the wonder of your body. It is in a constant dance to care for you. This system works, but sometimes too well, and especially if the world has worked against you for far too long and put you in a chronically stressed state. Then, not only is your brain's capacity to see the good and form new pathways more challenging, but you are also more likely to remember bad memories over nurturing ones. This is not your fault. It is the spiral of your nervous system's habitual and protective patterns, not a failing of you as a human.

Relaxation exercises prompt the vagus nerve to calm your heart and body. This was the simpler explanation I learned in medical school, but it's more nuanced science than that. Stephen Porges, who developed the *polyvagal theory*, describes the systems as a hierarchal ladder in your body.

The most evolved part of your nervous system is the *ventral (front) vagus complex*, the part of your vagus nerve that connects to the organs above your diaphragm, heart, lungs, face, and throat. It's your *front facing* to this world...how you send love, connect to and communicate with your voice and facial gestures, how you open your heart. In essence, it's how you find safety in your environment and, as well, in your own body when the world is not generous with it.

Next on the ladder is the sympathetic system that keeps you alert and confident but also mobilizes you to fight or flee in the face of a stressor. It's how you feel hypervigilant, on edge, anxious, or even fearful. It is your necessary defense system against threat.

The bottom of the ladder contains the most ancient component of your nervous system, the *dorsal (back) vagus complex*, the part of the vagus nerve that controls the organs below your diaphragm and lungs. It is how you immobilize if whatever you are facing is too much to manage at any one time, the way an animal might freeze in the wild as it faces a daunting predator. I think of it as having my back, literally, in that it operates essential functions for survival without my supervision.

I like to think of these three parts of the nervous system as a circle rather than a ladder, because they are always communicating and trying to achieve balance. If you feel loving, trusting, and safe, your *ventral vagus* is working well and keeps the other two defense systems gently in check. *It's okay, I'm okay, you can stand down.* That is aptly referred to as the *vagal brake* because, when it is stimulated, it inhibits the other two systems to achieve balance and ease in your body.

If you sense a risk or danger, the sympathetic nervous system may engage to mobilize you to fight or flee. *I need to get out of here.* If you cannot escape because the trauma or pain is too big to avoid, the *dorsal vagus* may kick in and try to save you by shutting down. You may literally pass out or more commonly numb or dissociate to withstand the pain. This can also manifest as a sense of hopelessness or withdrawal. Your body is literally trying to survive.

Take a Pause

Let's normalize body sensations you may encounter on this path to Justice and liberation. If your dorsal vagus has protected you to be in a shut-down or numb state, some of the exercises in the book may move you first in the circle to your sympathetic system and you may feel a jittery anxiety or hypervigilance before any calm. This is normal physiology. I think of this science in the body as a metaphor—as an uncomfortable untangling of the knots of our deepest inner wisdom that knew how to protect us but persisted for a bit too long. I also think of this discomfort as the kind that is inevitable with growing beyond the familiar, no matter how challenging that familiar has become. In Part 2, we will explore some techniques that help you attend to these bodily sensations. But this is also why you may want to reach out to a skilled therapist as you guide yourself on this path. From the beginning of time, we have healed most powerfully in community with others.

Remember I told you about my hypervigilance. That is not only consciously using my senses to look for or even smell danger. Your brain also literally scans the environment without you even realizing it, a process called *neuroception* that happens beyond rational thought. And even more amazingly to me, your brain constantly scans your body for signals as well, *interoceptive awareness*, looking for those Spidey senses and gut feelings. Your brain is constantly and delicately surveying your outer and inner landscapes to protect you. So, whatever bodily sensation emerged when that man threatened to kill my father (for me, it was my throat falling into my chest) is remembered as a cue of when not to trust.

The science shows that when you perceive unfairness in life, whether it was directed to you, another individual, or community, you generate a threat response in the brain and body that overstimulates your limbic system, your brain's emotional control center. Your body intakes this injustice as a danger because it is. But when you feel Justice, you release neurotransmitters of reward, such as dopamine and also oxytocin, the hormone of connection and safety. If you do not feel that the world around you is just, your commitment to Joy can create your own slice of Justice in this world, right inside your body.

You can also feel a bodily threat from not feeling that you belong in an environment or because of discrimination of any kind. Think about what happens in your body when you are in a workplace with no one who looks like you or a classroom where all the examples of success are from one homogenous group. Where do you fit in? Your body receives this pain of social exclusion in the same brain circuits as physical pain. They both hurt and are registered in your scanning as a threat.

Take a Pause

As we talk about Joy, realize that you may not feel as deserving of Joy if you don't see people who look like you practice it as well. So, give yourself the Justice of looking in your community, both in public figures as well as locally, for those who practice Joy in the face of challenge. Find role models and learn from them often.

I admit the inclination to engage with the world that beat you down may feel like the least desirable task. But when the ventral vagus is nourished, you are in your greatest balance and most loving, trusting state with not only the world but with yourself. This system keeps you feeling safe and seeing the world as safe to be in. Your body's capacity to flow more freely between these intricate systems of hypervigilance and trust will be your Justice.

POSITIVITY IS DANGEROUS

I will not tell you that everything will be okay or that if you stay positive, *you* will be okay. The truth is I can guarantee neither. The key (easier said than done) is to learn not to be overwhelmed by emotions as you recognize them, and we will untangle more about that in Part 2.

For now, it's worth saying that if anyone tells you to *Look on the bright side* or *Find the silver lining* when you're unable or unwilling to do so, that feels toxic because it is. They aren't seeing you fully. You aren't being validated and that's infuriating and even more inciting to your already-on-high-alert nervous system. The anger and pain from feeling invisible can put you in that *fight-or-flight* state, that revved-up sensation. Your body is in the mode of hearing those words as *danger* (remember, it's primed to see any threat) and it wants to fight back, flee, or freeze in your tracks. And now your nervous system is not only hypervigilant from the pain or loss itself but also by the attempts of others to dismiss it. The bigger problem is that if they don't see you, you may not see yourself either.

When your emotions are validated by yourself or others, as true, necessary, and normal, your entire nervous system can settle a bit more. What if your anger, for example, is the exact catalyst you need to metabolize your pain, and as such, is not something to avoid or *get over* but instead a part of you to acknowledge and honor?

You can and need to express your emotions; they all are necessary. Even challenging ones can create safety in your body if validated with love, by yourself and others. When you feel connected and trusted, your ventral vagus nerve can do its job to make you feel safe and comforted in the moment. And that's a critical step on the journey to Joy.

There was a time when my parents would ask me how Zubin was doing but not how *I was doing about* Zubin. Then, it got more awkward when they would ask Steve in private how he was doing and how things were *going for me*. I asked them why they avoided talking to me directly.

Their answer was enlightening and came from a place of compassion. *If you're feeling bad, we don't want to make it worse, and if you're feeling good, we don't want to bring you down.*

But when I'm facing pain, I am thinking about it most of the time. It may not be weighing me down constantly but it's in my psyche. Avoiding it felt like they were avoiding me. When they understood that, I felt seen. I had good friends and even close family members who never called me after Zubin's diagnosis, so they would not have to face the conversation. When I confronted them about this, they admitted they had consciously ignored me.

I couldn't face that pain.

I just didn't know what to say.

How about *I love you... no matter what?*

Sometimes, it's that simple.

If ignoring others is not the answer, then please don't ignore yourself. Ever. You deserve more than fleeing your precious, wise emotions. I know it's uncomfortable, even downright brutal. But, trust me, it's almost never a pain as enduring as the one you are running away from. You picked up this book because you want Justice, and the first step to that is liberating your own body by feeling what you feel and staying true to yourself. Every emotion is a stepping-stone to your potential transformation.

When you see yourself fully, you can then access your own wisdom that lies underneath all the pain... the deep inner wisdom that knows you can do this, that you can, *and were always meant to,* thrive and flourish.

PRACTICE: TOUCHING YOUR EMOTIONS

The practice of being with your emotions fully is a lifetime one. But let's start to deepen that journey with a simple exercise.

1. If you can, get quiet and bring attention to your breath; that helps bring attention into your body. This can be in a sitting, lying, or moving posture.
2. If you're able to do so, close your eyes, but if this does not feel safe, try to either fix them on a point or object ahead or gaze downward. Both of these start to bring your attention away from external distractions.
3. And then as you breathe in and out, just notice what you feel in your body, whether it be sensations, tension or ease, or emotions. With anything, acknowledge it and then return to your breath, over and over.
4. If emotions arise as you do this, you can merely name them as if you are lightly touching them and then return to your breath. Anger…breath…anger…breath…frustration…breath…and so on.
5. I practice this type of *touching* my emotions so that in any moment, I can do an on-the-spot exercise. Day-to-day, sometimes I will feel an emotion and just *touch* it as it is happening in real life. There's anger, I see you…breath…and so on.
6. This practice of visiting your emotions does not erase them (that is not the point) or even make them easier all the time. But it allows you to *see* and *touch* your emotions as guests that visit each day. When you do this, over time, you create

some space between you and the emotion so you can see or feel it more clearly. And most important, you affirm your emotions as part, but not all, of you.

DON'T BELIEVE THEIR LIES

Them: *God gives the greatest pain only to those who are spiritually strong enough to handle it.*

Me (in my head): *Fuck you, then I wish I was a spiritual sapling.*

But instead, I would nod and try to feign a smile.

Believe me, part of me wanted to desperately believe there was some truth in this platitude, so I could justify what had happened to Zubin. A reason, something supernatural, or even something I did wrong, anything. But your body always tells the truth when it recoils from saccharine lies.

Them: *I can't imagine...*

Me (in my head): *Lucky for you, you don't have to. Go on ahead with your more perfect life and I'll live this shitty one over here.*

But again, I would just nod and try to smile, and muster everything I could to stand there and be polite.

Take a Pause

I would make a plea to those who use the "I cannot imagine..." phrase. I encourage you instead to always imagine what it could be like to feel another's pain, not because you can know without walking their path, but because not trying to imagine, in my humble opinion, is a direct avoidance of empathy and connection that will separate you from them even more. Yes, their pain is so devastating that you don't even want to conceive of it and saying you can imagine anyone's exact pain is false and trite. Yet, being willing to step into this pain with them is a gift to both of you. It is the exact bridge you need to then be able to truly sit with your own pain when it comes your way. *I can't know what you are going through but I want you to know I am ready to sit here and be with you in it.* Build bridges of imagination every chance you get.

On and on it went in those first few months. Until people stopped visiting or calling. No more candles, casseroles, or cards. I don't know which was worse. Feeling more alone or their affirmations that Joy was not mine to have.

My life isn't nearly as tragic as many in this world. It's neither the easiest nor even close to the most trying. Searing pain comes to all of us, in differently sized packages. You can't compare pain and suffering. The grooves they carve within you are your own unique heart-print and only you can feel their depths. And the truth is that both physical and emotional pain are mysterious and dependent on a multitude of systems of privilege in this world. How much support and connection you have, whether your basic needs are being met, the stress of walking through this world if you are part of a marginalized* community, all these and more

* There is debate on the use of the term *marginalized* versus one like *historically excluded* and the consensus is not clear. I recognize that ongoing discussion; I chose to use *marginalized* here as a widely recognized descriptor of communities pushed to the margins of societal privilege and who carry a higher level of stress than those who are privileged in society.

combine to heighten or dampen pain. How it feels to you is the only thing that matters.

How is it that you aren't doubled over in disabling, excruciating pain every month? The surgeon pointed in disbelief to pictures of my ovaries tethered to the back of my abdomen in weblike, multilayered adhesions. He had just taken tumor-size growths off my ovaries for what we finally knew then was endometriosis and he was astonished that I had hardly mentioned the symptom of pain, a landmark sign of this condition. This had instead been part of an infertility workup and I was too preoccupied with the emotional pain of not having children. The truth is that my periods were always incredibly painful, the kind that double you over on the ground into a fetal position. I had adapted to and worked around them. But they also weren't as painful as these pictures suggested. I had support, love, food on the table, and meaning in my work; likely, those softened my pain. And yet, some people who share those privileges still feel it more intensely. Yes, pain remains a mystery. But it's always yours to unravel.

The human path through pain is universal, no matter how different it looks. Judging the value of your suffering just gives it more power. This book is about you taking yours back.

Joy is waiting for you, if you choose her. I swear, double-pinkie swear.

I now say, on the daily, that my life is perfect, not despite Zubin, but because of him.

No, not because *it happened for a reason* (I don't believe that lie either), not because *it's the best thing that happened to me* (I wouldn't wish this pain for any mother), but because it happened and there was no way to change that truth. And then I learned to keep my eyes and heart open.

My life is perfect because now I walk into it instead of away. Because I see that every step toward Joy is part of my revolution.

CHAPTER 3

The Present Moment Is Not Enough

THE PAST AND FUTURE MATTER TOO

I called it HBP, said Jade. That made sense since she dialogued with her high blood pressure. She was doing the same writing exercise as Maxine, but this time, my small group was in Minneapolis, in the aftermath of the murder of George Floyd. The city was reeling from the tragedy, and racial justice activists like Jade were exhausted from protests and tending to their community, yet again. She had come into the training feeling depleted, not only because of all the work demanded of her, but because the unrelenting fight for the safety of her community had started to feel so weighty that her hope had diminished.

Jade had offered to read her writing. The beginning of her inquiry into her high blood pressure was almost matter-of-fact, exploring how her younger body could have a condition usually ascribed to a more elder individual. How could these stiffened and hardened vessels arise in her still flexible and active body? But midway into the written conversation, *HBP* morphed into *high Black pressure* and that's when the aha moments and Justice began to unfold.

Jade saw that maybe *HBP* is so prevalent in her community not because her *body is flawed* but because she is a Black woman in America and she and her ancestors have had to endure the unyielding toll of racism in this flawed country. As her questions to *HBP* continued, she gained respect for her body and humility to be able to receive its powerful message.

I am done asking where you come from and want to know instead how to take back our power, she asserted now.

Jade had entered her body fully by asking, *What message does my body have for me?* She listened deeply and wrote, without letting her mind edit the answers. By the end of the writing, she was armed with the mission of taking this knowledge to her community. That afternoon, she won back a piece of power taken from her ancestors long ago. She returned to the past, acknowledged its pain, unlayered hers, and then harnessed hope for tomorrow. There are times when the today is too difficult to inhabit, and the past and future hold power that can soften the living in the present.

What if the present moment is sometimes *too small* a sliver? I teach mindfulness and meditation and deeply understand their power. I know that everywhere you turn, the teaching is that happiness or the absence of suffering are predicated on staying in the present moment. This is wisdom.... And I also get that at times, it's not enough. Not if we want Justice.

In Part 2, we will work with the tool of deep present moment awareness and when it's absolutely useful. But right now, I want you to understand why if we focus only on the present, we may miss powerful ways to unearth the Justice that has always lived in your body. And that deep cultivation may be exactly what you can give future generations.

That Justice is called *epigenetics*, a fancy word for the science of how our entire human genome is expressed. It's why your DNA is not your destiny but rather just the blueprint. You get to decide how the design emerges. Every cell in your body has the code to differentiate into whatever it will become: skin, liver, heart. But it's not just the cell that has this power; your environment can also impact this code. Whatever you eat, drink, however you move, think, or act in this world all determine how these cards play out. *You* get a say in how this blueprint gets expressed. It is a bigger story than we knew before. As I'm writing this book, a new study showed that people could reverse their biological age by three and a half years with just food and lifestyle, and by the time you are reading this, I'm guessing we will understand even more.

DNA exists in a double coil, but it is expressed through RNA, a messenger molecule that delivers the instructions to other cells. DNA can send different messages about cell activity based on your lifestyle. But this power also has challenges. Because *everything* you experience determines this design: racism, discrimination, trauma, all the shit you didn't ask for.

So, if you're a Black woman experiencing high stress—which, let's be real, every Black woman does just by moving in this white-male dominated world—then when you're pregnant, your child can suffer some of the effects of that high stress and the high cortisol that your body is putting out. If you've experienced a large-scale trauma, as my parents did during the Partition of

India or as families in the Holocaust, your children, and even grandchildren, can experience some of the effects of that trauma on their DNA.

Rachel Yehuda has shown in studies on Holocaust survivors and their families that these epigenetic changes, new markers on their DNA, can be passed down for at least two generations. These protein coatings that change the instructions caused higher stress and vulnerability in their children because of what the parents went through.

Take a Pause

These epigenetic changes may not only be a heritable legacy of the trauma but also a potential marker of their perseverance. The *deep knowing* of the cells that they have been persecuted possibly prepares future generations to be more vigilant.

Some argued that maybe parents passed down the trauma in their stories, but subsequent research has confirmed the actual genetic marker changes on the cells. And to me, even more amazingly, in 2013, a study showed that mice who were given a strong odor to smell paired with an electric shock passed an aversion to that odor to their naive adult children and grandchildren. This aversion was present even without the accompanying traumatic shock, just if the odor alone was presented to the future generations! The fear of that smell had *lived on* in the body. In addition, the odor had been presented to the original mice before conception of those offspring and did not happen with fostered children, so environment was not the culprit. *Trauma affects the family tree.*

I still feel amazed every time I say that. The things that *happen to* us change us, and possibly our entire lineage. We have language of that wisdom deep within us. *I'm not the same person anymore,* we say after a devastating experience. What you *perceive, feel, and do* about the things that happen to you change you as well. This explains why your fears or aversions may have something to do with an event you did not even experience yourself. I often think of this when I get curious about my heightened fear in the world. My father has relayed to us countless times the clear and brutal memories he still has of seeing dead bodies piled up on trains as he and his family fled Pakistan for India in 1947. What lack of safety did that experience plant in a young child? How did that change how he perceived the world? And has that shaped how my DNA has told me to be careful as I walk through mine?

It made sense then, at this same national training, when Kayla, a young Indigenous woman, asked, in the larger group, with tears in her eyes, *If I can mitigate some of this trauma in my body, can I heal the children and grandchildren to come?* All our hearts opened at the exact same moment in response to that question. She was really asking, *Is there any hope for those who come after me?*

That word *epigenetics* literally means "on top of genetics" (as in the way you eat, think, move, or worry is layered onto your DNA). Everything we experience takes on its own biology. So, yes, Kayla can do breathwork or meditation, for example, and manage her stress in a way that folds or unfolds these proteins.

And it's more nuanced and powerful than it sounds, more than just a breath. It's her capacity to breathe through a moment of pain or suffering in the present moment so that she can recognize that, no matter what has happened to her, she has the capacity to now give herself a moment of nurturing ease. How she turns genes on and off can change how her future children and grandchildren may respond to stress. She can hold the understanding that her today impacts their tomorrow. And holding that understanding helps her stay on her path to Justice. Her epigenome, the DNA story she writes, is in essence her personal biological Justice.

I also believe in the reverse, which is that when you find Joy and Justice in your body, you can heal those who came before you. Yes, those who have already walked through the fire. The past holds powerful messages for us. Of course, this is not something we can study through science, but maybe even more powerfully, we can experience it directly, in our lives.

COOKIE IS HIS NAME

My *bhua-ji*, my father's older sister, or bhuji as I called her, had one son. Her family of three lived in Pennsylvania. That was the story I knew. But underneath that was another one.

My bhuji had another child, an older son nicknamed Cookie. He died when he was about ten, before his brother, my cousin, or I were even born. I don't even have concrete memory of when or how I learned of Cookie, or even if anyone wanted me to know. I know that I was young enough to understand he couldn't walk, but old enough to wonder why no one could explain the reason. Anytime I asked about him, I was told that he was carried everywhere. Otherwise, no one talked about him. No one could explain to me how he died. It was as if everyone had forgotten him, or at least appeared to. No pictures (to this day, I have not seen one), no shared memories or stories (to this day, I don't know his real name), no mention of him in my bhuji's home, ever.

Implied to my young mind, but never said, was that Cookie was a *waste*, a life not worth speaking of because he only brought pain and suffering. That story came back to haunt me when Zubin was diagnosed. I instantly thought of Cookie after so very long. First, because I wanted to know if Cookie had DMD as I waited for genetic testing for our older son and myself. I feared our cultural ritual of secret keeping had endangered our genetic story in ways no one could have imagined. Zubin's genetic mutation turned out to be spontaneous, a sheer act of fate.

But since I had started thinking about Cookie, I couldn't stop. I thought about my bhuji who had lived out a kind of suffering that I now would get to know all too well. And so, when I cried about Zubin, I cried also for that cousin I never met. Not only for him, but also for me. Because forgetting him meant we could forget Zubin, and then by association, me. That our story could one day be discarded. That this all could be a waste.

Then, it made more sense to me that my bhuji was always somewhat gloomy. I felt it as a heaviness in my body when I was with her. And that whatever had happened to her for that decade in India was so dark and heavy that no one wanted her to relive it again. Maybe no one wanted to make her feel worse the way my parents worried about that for me. But I realize now that was too small a story for her. It's not that she wasn't able to be Joyful. It's that no one invited her to reclaim space for Joy and deep sadness to live together. Everywhere she turned, she was expected to push her suffering down and run away.

Now, I understand she could have lived a bigger story. I am certain she had always been able to both grieve Cookie *and* find Joy in this life. But maybe she mistakenly waited for permission to do so. I'm here to tell you not to wait. You don't need anyone else's permission: this is Justice you deserve, now.

Even in my first sorrowful days, I didn't want to cover my newly growing family in the shadow of my grief, but that didn't mean that I didn't acknowledge how heavy it felt. We needed to walk with, not under, its dark cloud. That included honoring Cookie as a forgotten soul who I would now remember and speak about so that his life wasn't lost. And look, here is his story now for all to know. (I literally can't see through my tears as I write that.)

I wish my bhuji were here to read this book, so I could tell her I now see the complexities of her struggle, not only the struggle with pain that everyone highlighted, but also her struggle to make space for Joy. Cookie could have been her catalyst. I wish she were here so I could tell her that I am reclaiming our family's past as a way to live out my present. I redeem Cookie's story that I myself needed to acknowledge and grieve. He's not a waste, he's not forgotten. He's a story worth remembering. And you likely have one too.

Take a Pause

On this path, if you acknowledge past stories that have restricted your present capacity to expand into Joy, you can eventually rewrite them and envision a different future for yourself. Do you have a Cookie or another story that has been told or kept from you in shameful whispers and has unconsciously informed how you believe or don't believe in your capacity for Joy?

WE ARE ALL ABLE

Sometimes the baggage of your past can't just be put down or unpacked. It needs to be incinerated. In my language, there is a term, *bechaara*. I don't even know what the equivalent in English would be. Even saying *poor thing* is too understated. It's far beyond that, a term used anytime someone's life has fallen below what anyone else would want and denotes a kind of wasted-ness. A sense that there is no hope. Having a child like Zubin has meant that I have heard that term far too many times, from the streets of India to community gatherings.

This has even come from some members of my own wide, extended family who don't know how to negotiate his value in their mind. I admit, not everyone is like this exactly all the time and many family members defy this description. But this generalization holds in the same way racial bias does. You are given it and then must deny or work against it.

My cultural community's story reinforced this belief of one's value only more. At every gathering, the uncles and aunties asked only about success and otherwise, a shameful silence fell. How could a disabled life be valuable if you are destined to never have a job (and produce), go to college (so that you can produce), or succeed (produce money and assets)?

It's not just my South Asian culture. The American culture that I grew up in painted a story that filled my psyche. Growing up, any child with a disability was put in a different classroom; hell, I'm not even sure where they were because I never saw any. Disabled children were in different rooms, buildings. Different worlds.

My husband says in his school, disabled children were called the "B-9'ers" because they were in building B, room 9. Steve never interacted with them but sometimes he would see them going out to play in their own space or to their separate bathroom or eating area. He tells me the term *B-9'ers* became a way to degrade or tease other kids on the playground. We can tell ourselves that giving disabled kids separate space, so they would get more attention or their needs served better, started as a compassionate decision. But the studies clearly show that not only disabled children, but *all* children do better academically when they're together. And I think, more important, children have less prejudice if they are in classrooms together. If they are taught difference needs to be separated and that some lives are not valuable enough to be in the same room, what kind of society and leaders are we creating?

So, put all this together and imagine the unconscious limiting stories in my mind when trying to advocate for my son's inclusion in the schools. When trying to hold Joy in the face of all the stories I've been told and shown. It was some seriously heavy baggage to put down.

I had to wade through all that deep shit and see my own darkness. Admit that maybe I, too, didn't value his life as much as I wanted to. That maybe I saw him as being in a different world. Having a different worth. Years later, it's still hard to admit I thought, no not just thought—I believed—all that. That's the story I had been given and I had held on to it.

Now I rewrite that bechaara story. But it took serious and deep, inner work and the first step was seeing my baggage in the first place. Seeing it in my own heart and admitting that just because it lived there didn't mean it was right or that I was inherently bad. It was time to unlearn and relearn a different way.

Take a Pause

Where in your own life do you need to see better? Trust me, until you see the mess, you can't wade past it. You don't have to fully untangle all of it to start the journey to Joy. If you can just see it, catch a glimpse to start, and maybe admit it, then much of it can happen in parallel to what we will do together. Justice will prevail if you take this step on your way to Joy. But you can't walk the path if you're blocked by dirty suitcases.

An Indigenous spiritual mentor once explained to my friend that in scary, hard places, she must remember, *there is a featherbed on the other side.* Now, I can't promise light, soft feathers all the time, but I think he meant that if you do the work, even start the work, you'll have a reward on the other side of that. I choose to trust we all have a soft featherbed awaiting us for a moment of rest any time we need it on the journey.

CHAPTER 4

Your Body Knows

AND IT REMEMBERS

In December 2020, I was one of the US frontline health-care workers who received the first waves of the COVID-19 vaccine. As the needle went into my arm, I felt pure awe. Both that I was receiving this gift and that it had been created so swiftly in what felt like an unimaginable scientific miracle. As I waited in the jubilant observation room with my colleagues' mix of anxiety and honor to be the guinea pigs, I found silent space. I was so overwhelmed with gratitude for this vaccine, for my body, and for this privilege that I needed to close my eyes and linger in the moment. When I look at the picture of myself right after the vaccine, all those emotions rush back as if they have never left their intangible home just beneath the surface of my skin.

When I returned for my second vaccine a few weeks later, I remained in awe but felt more nonchalant. I joined my colleagues in the large observation room, smiled and exchanged some pleasantries, and then sat down to text my son who had chauffeured me that night and was waiting outside the hospital. *I will be out soon, I don't even know if I will wait the entire 15 minutes.* So confident was I in that moment. And then in less than five minutes after the vaccine entering my arm, I started to feel something I had never felt before. A scratchy feeling and then tightening in my throat. I found a monitoring nurse in the room and after explaining my concern, she carefully observed me. The sensation only got stronger, and our next move was to swiftly visit the emergency room. My fear mounted. She called my husband for me because by the time we reached our destination, I could not muster the breath to speak. Thankfully, I had a good outcome and for all intents and purposes, the scary evening eventually ended, but only in my mind. My body still held on.

In the next several months, I had three instances of that same tightening sensation in my throat, two intense and scary enough to call 911. Each time was after ingesting nuts, a food I had eaten my entire life. All three times, my symptoms resolved after reassurance, precautionary allergy medication, and deep breathing. You may wonder why the reaction persisted and with nuts when the initial time I felt this was with a needle, not from a morsel in my mouth.

We will never know the reason for sure or have a laboratory test to give us an answer. But I do have a theory that comes not only from two and a half decades of caring for patients with panic and anxiety but most important, from deep listening to my body's wisdom. That night of the second vaccine, my sensation of a closing throat and gasping for air was very real. I had no conscious fear of an adverse reaction, despite experiences of caring for patients with this challenge and living the anxiety of it as a mother.

The fear in those gasping-for-air moments may have untangled my decade-plus of hypervigilant fear for Zubin's life-threatening allergies to nuts. Surveying every food at a birthday or dinner party, obsessively reading every label, all this was my normal life activity. And then that night in the emergency room, my body felt the exact sensation I had avoided so long for him. Each time my body then ingested nuts, they were not only a food but a reminder of what I had held on to for so long. My body sent me a message of remembered panic, in the most primal, ancient way it knows. It reminded me, *You have been scared for far too long and it has taken a toll.*

I still remember a time, well over a decade ago, when I had severe and persistent tingling sensations in my arms and the neurologist ordered an MRI of my head and neck to look for multiple sclerosis. I was the right age, gender, and symptom profile for what the textbooks describe. My mind was frantic thinking of the ramifications this kind of diagnosis could have in our already stretched household. I spoke to an Integrative Medicine mentor of mine the day before the test and she simply asked me, *Tanmeet, what do you think your nerves are telling you?* And then she drew what seems now an obvious parallel between my symptoms and my stress over the neurologic disease of my son. The body knows and always speaks the truth.

It's not every day (in fact there was only this one) that I open the exam room door to see a woman with a shaved head, in a maroon flowing robe with saffron edges. I was a bit taken aback but settled into my seat alongside her. *This should be interesting.*

Dina, a middle-aged white woman, was a new patient. A Buddhist nun, she had lived in an ashram outside the US for the last twenty years. *Oh, okay, she's the real deal,* I thought.

Flank pain had impacted her for the past month, intermittently but daily, and of enough severity that she was restricted in how much she could sit in meditation or contribute to the daily chores of her *sangha* (spiritual community). It was starting to cause her some significant stress, and now she was unable to just *work through it.*

Along with a usual medical history, recounting the pain, its nature, and associated symptoms, I heard about her transition to nonmonastic life. She admitted this had been hectic as she had loads of paperwork to fill out to be reacclimated into society and receive health insurance and social security benefits, not to mention adjusting to the two decades of changes in technology and culture.

I did a thorough exam that did not reveal anything out of the ordinary other than the location of the pain, and I offered some diagnostic work to start the investigation process. She was visibly disappointed when she came back in a week and received all normal lab results. I then offered some diagnostic imaging to take the evaluation further. By this point, her pain had actually worsened, and I worried there might be something larger going on.

Fortunately, the imaging was all normal, but she found this information disappointing as there was still no identifiable source for her discomfort. We agreed she would return in a week and I would brainstorm some more. Up until her appointment, I went through all the diagnostic possibilities and wondered whether I had missed something. And I had. She was so certain there was a physical source, some medical pathology to blame for her pain, that I, too, had become preoccupied with her fear.

I felt incredibly anxious to suggest to a practicing nun that stress might be the culprit, but that was my task. When she came in, I presented my thought process and then the ways that stress can inhabit the body in physical symptoms. I suggested that we look over her self-care practice and see whether we could optimize it, feeling way out of my league to do a meditation prescription for a Buddhist nun! But she was gracious and agreed to try. (Her pain did improve and in not too long a time frame.)

When my patients ask me about seemingly unexplainable sensations that defy every workup and test for a tangible answer—*Dr. Sethi, why can't anyone give me a diagnosis?*—I tell them what I told Dina and what I *do* know to be true:

What your mind and heart cannot resolve, your body will hold on to.

PAIN IS WISE

In the days after Zubin's diagnosis, in one of the many phone calls with my parents, trying to make sense of this new life I had been given, I heard something that stirred my revolution. I was recounting Zubin's struggles from the very beginning. He had come out crying at birth, but then very quickly, the delivery room fell silent, including him. I heard, *He's blue!* (I knew, even in my postdelivery haze, that he had stopped breathing.) A team quickly arrived to intubate him. Zubin was in the NICU for eleven long days and recovered slowly. But we had almost lost him in those fragile seconds after birth and I naively thought then that he had overcome his biggest challenge.

It would have been better if he had died then, I remember my father saying wistfully.

I know now that my father meant that with compassion, that his early death would have been easier for me than the prolonged one that awaited him now. But it was one of those moments you want to rewind. *Please, take that back.* And I had nothing to say in return. My heart was shattered. Even though I wanted to cry or scream, I just sat silently, trying to hold what was left of those pieces. Worse yet, maybe he was right. Maybe he only reflected the worst of what I wished for my broken Mama heart.

That was one of the two times in those fragile, raw days that, along with the pain, I also felt a surge of energy in my broken heart. A sensation of something different. It wasn't yet a surge of Joy, but one of resistance. Of my revolution in its infancy. The kind that swells up when you are rejected unjustly. The kind where your body tells you that this is not okay even when your mind absorbs the untruths you are given. Your body is wise and tells you the truth even if you can't translate it in that moment.

In that instant and the many instants after, despite the intense grief, what I felt in my body was a deep knowing that I didn't want Zubin to be forgotten or pushed to the side. I didn't want him better off dead. I thought then that the sensation I felt in my chest was deep hurt or anger, but later, I realized that physical pain represented much more. I was birthing my revolution inside of me right then and there. I was pushing against the fiery edge of that pain. And I might have missed all that if I had not learned to stop turning away from it. Or if I had channeled it into an unnecessary blaming of my father for his words.

Take a Pause

You have embodied wisdom in how you describe pain. You feel *heavy hearted* or your stomach is *in knots* or *full of butterflies.* You know things in your heart and gut brain and yet you all too often dismiss your body when it tries to communicate with you. Your body carries it all, the pain, as well as the unique capacity to untangle it. So, if you're feeling stuck, frustrated, or exhausted, you're in the right place. You're in your body and that's where the magic can unfold. Not outside, not from anywhere but yourself. In Eastern and yogic philosophies, the description of the *subtle body* is used to explain its powerful potential to be the vessel of awakening if we can stay alert to its energies or messages.

If you get really quiet and listen, the kind of quiet where you sometimes first have to wade through a sea of pain that you never asked for, you'll hear the hushed whispers in your body that ask, almost plead, to heal.

I naively thought Cookie's death didn't have a huge impact on me before my own son's diagnosis. After all, it wasn't *my* brother who died. It wasn't *my* mom who was sad. It was just a tragic family story. But it had not only affected me, it lived within me, taking up dark space. Most family trauma does, even when we think it's *not ours*. And now, it had the chance to well up in my own waves of grief as a piece of me that had needed healing all along.

I now know that baggage was wounding so many.

My father who later revealed the underlying pain that likely lay behind what he said.

My cousin who later admitted to me that his family of three lived in the dark shroud of shame cast by Cookie's shadow.

Me because Cookie lived in my body as a shameful secret.

Today, I am so very thankful for what my father said and for my surge of resistance. I'm so grateful he bravely voiced his pain. Without his, I wouldn't have felt mine and tended to my own wound that needed so much care.

That wound has taught me so very much, not only about my baggage and my grief for Zubin, but also about the fierce need for all of us to eventually turn toward our pain, even the kind that, in the moment, pierces our heart. The kind that makes us want to turn away and wish we had never received it.

After Zubin's diagnosis, nothing felt fair. Not the diagnosis or anyone's words. I wanted Justice, which I thought meant a different life. Or a cure. Now, I know that the Justice I wanted in that moment was always mine to have, in *this* life. Joy was—is—my act of resistance.

By practicing Joy, I have fought against this forgetting and hushed whispers.

I have accepted that my family and culture's beautiful tapestries also have murky patches that threaten my capacity for Joy.

I have erased the potential broken and unspoken family story that Zubin's life and my life or mothering of him are not worthy. I have erased the stories I was given so I could write my own.

PAIN MOVES

My father later explained to me that everyone encouraged his sister to put Cookie in a home for children who *had no future.* That sent shivers down my spine. As a young mother in India with a child who no one valued, she lived in a culture that must have made her feel *less than.* I told you the trauma was so great that she always walked with a shadow of deep sadness. My father must have been in pain, too, watching his sister, and may have felt sad now about the advice, which lived dormant for decades in his body, and then released in his words to me. Maybe his body had held on to them under the surface the whole time, until they found a way to move and heal in another story.

Now I look back at my bhuji and see the strength she must have had to simply endure. She defiantly carried Cookie everywhere and never gave in. She kept him in her own home where she felt he belonged. Her capacity for revolution was right there all that time and that resistance could have moved her to greater Joy.

My bhuji and I were close mostly only in that familial way. We really didn't have a relationship of more substance—until Zubin was diagnosed. Then, she called me every month, ostensibly to say hi, but she had never done that before in our lives. And she always asked about Zubin. And she always said in some way how she knew how hard it is, but that she was happy I was finding a way. Maybe she was reliving her suffering with someone who may finally get it. She would then anoint me at the end with Waheguru's blessings to be strong. It would go like that every time. I unfortunately never asked more. At the time, I didn't have the stamina to do so.

Finding my capacity for Joy in this life may also heal those who came before me. Walking through this life with Zubin while seeking unapologetic Joy showed my bhuji that it was possible. That I didn't have to play the part of the suffering mother. That I could hold all the pain and yet, also say my life is beautiful. She got to see some of that before she died.

My Joy in this life heals my father. He sees that it's a gift that Zubin survived. He sees his daughter soar and another way that life can be valued, no matter how short that life is. He tells me often how proud he is of me, and these words heal both of us.

My Joy in this life heals my cousin, Cookie's brother, who has told me repeatedly that seeing me live with Joy *despite the pain you have with Zubin* shows him there was, in fact, another way to do this. It reveals to him the possibilities that his parents couldn't live out for him.

If I can heal a part of my bhuji, my father, or my cousin, who's to say that I can't heal the ancestors I didn't even meet? I think about this every time I see Joy living in this world where one could not have predicted, amidst a legacy of suffering. We can't suddenly heal an entire world's history of wrongs. But every step, every action is one stride toward more Justice. One light footstep toward ancestors settling their souls a bit more peacefully. And your soul as well.

PAIN TEACHES

Remember I told you that I don't usually have cool animals or light-filled spirits visit me in any guided imagery? The first and rare time I did changed everything. A year after Zubin's diagnosis, I was in Minneapolis at the start of winter, the most unlikely setting in my mind for a life-altering experience.

I was attending the final certification training for the mind body medicine small group work I now do. On that day, the agenda included what is called a fishbowl exercise where the founder, Jim Gordon, MD, conducts a small mind body medicine skills group, the type we use in our work all over the world, but this time, in front of the whole group of attendees so that we can observe and hopefully glean some pearls of wisdom.

Imagine there are more than two hundred people sitting in a large room, chairs arranged in concentric rings around the open middle where there are eight chairs arranged in their own inner circle. Seven people from the training bravely volunteer to sit in this innermost space and participate in a small group in front of this large crowd.

I had been facilitating these groups for a couple of years by this point and the work had already sung to me as deep work of my heart. I was ready to soak up as much as I could, but here as I sat watching these individuals raise their hands to enter the circle, all I could think was, *No way would I do that.* I had observed this fishbowl before and had been struck by how raw and authentic the group was, even in this seemingly contrived setting. But I prefer to do my own soul growth without peering eyes and hearts, no matter how loving. As more hands raised, I heard a small voice somewhere within me saying, *Do it.*

Almost involuntarily, I muttered softly but out loud, *Maybe I should.* As if the voice I heard was now coming through me to make it more real. A faculty member, sitting next to me, heard my mumble, leaned closer, and said, *Do it. It will change your life.*

And just like that, as if moved by a puppeteer, my own hand went up just in time to be the last one chosen. Jim first asked why I wanted to be in the group. And before I could think about it, I said, *I want to learn how to live with fear.* In usual form, he answered, *Tell me more about that.*

And in that moment, it did not matter that hundreds of people were looking at me. I just looked at him, my voice quivering, and said, *My son is dying... and I am so scared.*

There was an instant moment in the room of weighted silence, the inaudible sound of chests heaving, eyes tearing, and then sighs being exhaled slowly enough to make space for what I just said. He invited me into the group.

We did a customary opening meditation of breathwork. We then each checked in and shared how we were feeling in that moment. There is always a skill to learn in a group session and on this day, Jim decided we would practice a wise guide meditation. It is an exercise practiced in many forms but all, in my estimation, are rooted in and borrowed from ancient Indigenous practices of going deeply inward to find wisdom from guides or possibly ancestors from your own inner soul's knowing.

You are led first into a guided imagery of a safe place of your creation and then afterward invited to see a *wise or special being* approach to whom you can ask questions or from whom you can get a message.

Even first-timers to this imagery somehow get messages from all kinds of amazing images. Animals, ancestors, light forms, you name it. But not me. I had always had a relaxing meditation and was able to access a safe place in my mind, but never a meaningful wise guide and it, frankly, always made me feel like I was missing out. (And even a little embarrassed when I would admit out loud to the group there was no guide in my imagery.)

So, here I was in the middle of this room in front of hundreds of participants and many of my teachers, and when Jim said this was the exercise he chose, my heart fell. (As an aside, he rarely chooses this exercise in the fishbowl, and I have never seen him do it since.)

Great, now I have to admit in front of everyone that I didn't see anything! That no guide came to give me sage advice. *Deep breaths, Tanmeet, deep breaths.* Maybe I could be a reassuring example for anyone who also had my same experience in the past. With that pacifying thought in my mind and heart, the imagery began.

Jim asked us to first imagine we were in a safe place. I automatically always go to the same one in my mind—a warm, tropical beach. That's my happiest place, where I feel like my soul can soar free. I'm never relaxed unless I'm guaranteed bright sun and blazing heat. And this time, I found myself at a creek along a wooded trail. I was jarred: *What the hell, it could be cool or even chilly in these woods.* But I heard him say, *Just relax into wherever your mind has gone.*

So, I soaked into this new place with all my senses.

I saw so many shades of green.

I felt the soft give of the forest floor beneath me as I gently explored.

I smelled the crisp needles of the trees.

I heard the babbling of the running creek and saw the light reflect off its stones in a way that allowed the sun to warm and reassure me that maybe this place was okay.

Jim invited us to see whether there was a wise or special guide appearing. (*Oh no, here we go,* I thought, *just when I was enjoying this. . . .*)

But just like that, for the first time ever, I saw another person in my imagery.

It was my Pashi Masi, my mom's closest ever cousin sister, her best friend in the entire world.

Masi is what we call our mother's sisters, shortened for the words meaning "just like mother." She had always been someone I resonated with deeply and had tragically passed away seven years prior. She was a magnet field therapist in India—the only healer I knew of in our family—so my only guidepost and a perennially loving figure. Every single time we left India, she cried as if it was the first time all over again.

There she was, sitting at the creek and then there I was laying my head in her lap with her stroking my hair. I could easily feel her soothing fingers along my scalp and I found myself immediately in tears as I lay there. Her comforting hand traveling from my head, down my neck, and through my long hair. And my tears flowed and flowed, offering my lips their salty stream.

Jim invited us to ask our guide a question and mine came without hesitation.

How am I going to do this, Masi?

And I knew she understood that by *this*, I meant how was I to live this nightmarish tragedy, this life I didn't want.

How am I going to do this?

Each time I asked, my tears flowed heavier.

You will do it, beti *(child)*, she reassured me, repeating the phrase like a mantra each time.

I was not satisfied.

I pressed her further. *But* how *will I live this life?*

Again, she reassured me. And again, I asked, hoping she could solve this pain for me.

Silence.

Hands through my hair.

Silence.

More tears.

Until she spoke.

Let Zubin teach you.

And then my tears flooded.

I was so solidly in this scene, this space of the creek, her hand. I could feel her caress. I could hear her voice.

Let him teach me.

It felt so simple, so obvious.

Let him teach me.

In an unknown space of time after this, I heard Jim's voice directing us back to the room. My eyes slowly, fearfully opened, not wanting to leave the safety and clarity of that moment, wanting it to be real and everlasting. I lifted my eyelids, and the creek and Masi were gone.

Just like that. All that was left were the very real tears in my mouth and running down my neck.

Jim asked everyone to share, if they were willing, what they experienced in the imagery.

When he got to me, at the very end of the circle, I looked at him, tears flowing down, and recounted it all. The creek, the lap, the hand, the question, and finally the answer.

Let Zubin teach you.

In that moment, as I looked at him, tears instantly streaming down his face, I felt all two hundred–plus hearts in that room connect and lock in what I can only describe as an invisible energetic string that held us all together as if our hearts opened at the same time and reached out for one another. Because we knew this answer was for all of us.

This moment was what people call life changing.

From that moment on, I did what Pashi Masi said. I let Zubin teach me.

And now he can teach you.

Not because Zubin is *your* teacher.

But because you have your own and you can listen.

CHAPTER 5

Rewrite the System

WHAT IS YOUR JOY?

I have wracked my brain to find a definition for Joy only to realize the obvious truth. That if I use one, then I am only subscribing to the same confines of a system that took it away from me. The first step in rewriting a system is for me to understand *my* own Joy. As it is for you to know yours.

You know your Joy when you feel it. Your body gives you signals that you have stepped into it. And one definition does not suffice. Allow yourself many possibilities.

Take a Pause

It may be easier to recognize this Joy when you have made space for it to grow. Stay with me through the end of Part 1. Take a pause, go back to any exercises that feel resonant. Spend time with this. There is no deadline to finding your Justice; it's always your exact right time.

For me, Joy is floating in warm ocean water or taking a walk in the trees. It's cooking and sharing a good meal. It's dancing my heart out. For my fiftieth birthday, I had a *bhangra* party and danced for hours with friends and family who had flown in to celebrate, but especially my teenage children. There were moments on that dance floor that I felt such intense Joy, it brought me to tears. I closed my eyes and thought, *Wrap this in a capsule and access it when you need it, Tanmeet. Remember this moment to carry yourself through others.* In that moment, I was doing what I love most with those I hold the most dear, feeling intense gratitude and awe. That all three of my children moved and sang Joyfully with me, that my son in a wheelchair was so free on the dance floor (and could outdance anyone there!), that I was surrounded by family I loved and community of all ages moving to the rhythms that my body feels most at home in.

I feel Joy when I work deeply with those in spiritual crisis and feel the seeds of their transformation. Not because I have *helped* them but because their potential inspires mine.

I feel Joy when I feel like I belong...in my workplace, in my community, in my home.

There are countless ways that I feel Joy, but in all of them, I know when I feel it in my body. I notice an expansive opening in my chest. A lightness in my heart space and an ease in my shoulders. And yes, the feeling is often ineffable, reminiscent of Rumi's words:

When you do things from your soul, you feel a river moving in you, a joy.

It is my river. And I know her well.

When things are going well, linger so you can access it again when needed. When you're having a beautiful, Joyful moment, go with it. Yes, it will be fleeting; all of life is. But feel it in every part of your body. The more you soak in that Joy, the more you signal neurochemicals like dopamine, as a reward, to then notice Joy as something to want *more* of.

PRACTICE: GET TO KNOW YOUR JOY

1. What is your Joy? When do you feel it? If you haven't had it in a long time, think back to when it was present, in what moments? What were you doing? And if you can't remember, imagine what it would feel like. Write it down, describe it with as many senses as possible, put it up on sticky notes where you can see it and believe you can have it. Maybe it's in a piece of art or a photograph. Make a Joy wall or space in your home where you can remind yourself regularly.
2. What does it feel like in your body and where do you feel it? Close your eyes and see whether you can access any of those sensations.
3. Use a journal, a voice recorder app, muse on it in your mind, move with it—whatever helps you recall your memories of Joy. Come back to this exercise often, especially if it was challenging. There is no timeline to your system, it is yours to write and rewrite.

CHARDI KALA

Every revolution deserves a good battle cry, such as a mantra or soothing phrase you can come back to to remind you of your path to Joy. I invite you to design your own, but I will also offer inspiration. Not because it is the *right* or *only* phrase, but because it is a powerful one that has withstood the test of time.

I offer this battle chant from my Sikh culture to yours. As inspiration from a people who have endured so much but still stand tall. We have called upon it through historical religious persecution since our birth as a faith in the 1400s in a dominant Hindu-Muslim land. Through the Partition of India, the genocide of our people in the 1980s, and the hate that still exists throughout the world for those who look and pray like us.

Through it all, we return to *Chardi Kala*, often translated in an underestimate as "eternal Joy" or "the absence of negativity." But it runs much deeper than this. It is instead the power to face whatever adversity comes your way and *still* find Joy, no matter what. It is a reminder that you always have that capacity to thrive. Often chanted as a true battle cry in history, I think of it as a call to Justice, here and now, in your body, in your life.

The choice is yours, to borrow and lovingly nurture this principle from Sikh culture as one of your own calls for Justice. This can be an ingredient in your path to Joy, or you can use it as inspiration to dig deep into your own ancestry or the global lineages for one that resonates for you. When you don't believe Joy is accessible, look for ways others in the world have accessed this power, even amid brutal struggles.

Take a Pause

I invite you to think of your ancestral circle as a wider one than you may usually conceive of. When I need to harness power that I cannot feel in my own body or spirit, I do a practice of calling on this circle. I think not only of ancestors in my own blood lineage, known and unknown to me. I call on the ancestors of my global lineage, knowing that the collective past holds power for all of us. Listen with your whole body for their messages.

NOT ALL OR NONE

After I give a talk, people come up to me and very often start with the same preface:

What you said really touched/inspired/moved me...

And then immediately:

But I just don't think I can do that...

The *that* refers to:

The gratitude

The compassion

The hope

The grace

The all of it.

It just feels too hard.

My response: *And how is what you're doing working for you?* 'Cause here's the truth: If you're feeling moved, it is because something I've said is calling to some deep part of you. Story is medicine. When you see the potential of your human capacity in another, you want to mimic that and possibly, even more important, you finally believe that potential must exist within you.

I can't make this easier. The act of finding Joy is hard work at first, no matter how I slice it. And the role of suffering and being the sufferer is ever looming and big in this world. But this is not the looming-over-you-impossible work either. This work is powerful resistance that eventually brings more ease. So, it's time for the talk.

Yes, your life is hard . . . and you can still find Joy to live with all that.

Yes, your emotions are real . . . and still you can have emotions of lightness and ease that live right next to them.

Yes, your story is painful . . . and it can also have meaning.

Your anger, your sadness, your fear, all of it, are necessary to find your Joy. Together they are your power.

Nothing in this world is binary. Not race, not gender, not emotions, and definitely not your story. Embrace a truth that allows the entirety of your life and all its complex nuances to come through. If you shut that out, your story will read only one way . . . impossible.

And this book is about you finding the possible.

You don't need to be strong or superhuman to find Joy.

You seek Joy to find your power.

YOUR OWN GROUND RULES

A belief is merely a thought repeated over and over. If you've convinced yourself Joy is not yours to have, it's time for a better road map. And, trust me, what you say to yourself makes a difference.

Science is catching up to what the ancient sages have known for far longer about mantra, Sanskrit for "mind" (*manas*) and "tool" (*tra*), used in every spiritual tradition known. When you remember your own personal Justice mantra, over and over, you turn down a part of the brain called the default mode network (DMN), a region referred to as the busy mind, full of ruminating thoughts on the past and future and related to self-judgment, a default way of thinking. Mantra brings you to a less noisy place where you can connect to something bigger outside yourself. It also doesn't matter whether you recite an ancient Sanskrit mantra, the Lord's Prayer, or any calming phrase to get these results. Especially if you hum or chant a mantra, you activate the ventral vagus, making you want to reengage with the world. So, sing them out loud!

I will share a few of my mantras on Joy, only to guide you to yours. They can be your point of departure or inspiration to find your beliefs, your new guideposts on this road map.

MY GROUND RULE:

Joy and happiness are not the same thing.

My infertility battle hollowed out my spirit. I spent night after night crying about my persistently negative white pregnancy sticks while I went to never-ending baby showers. It was torture, mustering happiness for my friends while I felt that my body was betraying me. Which only further cemented my internal dialogue that I was not worthy if I could not achieve this dream that seemed to come so easily to every woman I knew. And fake smiling while I answered the never-ending question, *When are you and Steve thinking of having kids?*

For God's sake, we weren't only thinking about it, we were overthinking it, planning sex under the luckiest full moons, charting our astrology if needed, doing any crazy diet anyone suggested, all that shit, all the time.

At one point, after I had cried for hours about yet another negative pregnancy test, Steve got home late from work to me on the couch in a puddle of tears. And I swear to you, I looked straight at him and asked, *Can I just make sure we have this right? Can we go over how babies are made?*

I swear, I as an adult *and* a physician who delivered babies, asked him this.

It was my last desperate plea to the universe that I must be missing something because none of this was fair. (He did assure me I had the process down, by the way.)

I felt betrayed by my body, by this life. If only I could have at least one child, I would finally be happy. When I did finally get pregnant years later, I was happy, no doubt. But I was not Joyful, truly. Because everything depended on the next thing I needed. The next child, the right job, always something.

I was getting happiness and Joy confused. I thought if the conditions were right, Joy would appear.

I have a *before* and *after* life. The *before* I gave birth to Zubin when everything at least looked more perfect and the *after* he was born, when I had the nagging feeling of something being gravely wrong. And then the big *after*, that fateful Monday when I found out I was right.

I was much happier in my *before* life, even in the face of past depression and life struggles. But I was never as Joyful as I am now. Never.

My happiness was always dependent on some *thing*. I was attached to outcome. And my mood was then attached to that. That's the kind of confused relationship I had with Joy. It seemed functional at the time, but it was quite one-sided. That wasn't a way for me to thrive.

MY GROUND RULE:

I deserve and choose Joy.

More than one thing can be true at the same time. This world, my life, can be unfair or difficult and I can still choose Joy to exist alongside all that.

This happens through work, not of the capitalist kind, but through the soul work we are doing together in this book. The kind that fuels every cell in your body, the kind that makes you want to do more. (Remember that dopamine!) The kind of work that, once you move into it, becomes an effortless flow, and then Joy starts to work on you.

Life proceeds at its own pace, doling out wins and, at other times when you least expect, heart-aching challenges. Along the way, somewhere, somehow, you decide life is either good or bad. You create and stick to a story that somehow the tragedies of this life hold power over you. At any one time, you can decide you're defeated or powerful, but you're writing that story based on what life gives to you instead of what you give to it.

The path isn't always easy. You may need to go slow and take long breaks. The best neuroplasticity happens in incremental pieces, so in fact, taking it slow is your body's deep knowing of how to do this. The path will often require added safety and love through community or professionals.

And even if you don't fully believe or trust me yet, if the path you're on isn't working well enough, it's time to give another one a spin.

Imagining what is possible is core to the work of being human. And maybe, just maybe, you'll find that Joy is not *because* of the work, it is *in* the work.

MY GROUND RULE:

Joy is real and always waiting for me.

Joy is as alive as it gets. Think: quantum physics meets powerful, flowing energy.

I've gotten over this lie that Joy is a *thing* that I can find, a mythical destination that I reach, and think of her instead as an alive companion.

Sometimes I repeat to myself

Joy is real. She's alive.

Like my own Justice mantra. On repeat until it becomes a part of my body's fabric.

Then, I bring in a sense of calm and safety through the ventral vagus nerve, and most important, I prioritize *my* story, not someone else's. It reminds me that this is a safe step toward my

Justice. Trust me, if it sounds silly to do this, silly is better than hopeless, any day of the week.

Take a Pause

When you imagine what you want in the future, you're more likely to reach your goal. Not only that, but even if you don't practice a skill, you can strengthen muscles by just imagining you are exercising them. Sit with that power. Putting the image in your brain paves the pathways so that it is easier to walk them when the opportunity arises. So, call in Joy however feels right to you. Whisper, shout it out, write it down, meditate on it. If this feels silly, know that people at the top of their game, from surgeons to pianists, have more success if they practice their skill while also mentally imagining the skill improving. Your imagination is your Justice.

Remember, people say to me: *I can see how it worked for you, but it feels too hard for me to do that.*

My other response: *It's just an invitation. An invitation to a different way to live this life.* That same offer awaits you now, here, in this book. This work will liberate you from the grip of pain so that you may feel much more—hope, Joy, peace. In other words, *not* doing the work will keep you in the spiral of whatever darkness you're swimming in now. This book is for everyone who has said, *I could never do that.* That's the mind trying to override what the body proves it can do every day: move forward, nurture, and heal. It only feels hard because you're in the habit of doing life a different way. But I promise, the Justice work of feeling fully and knowing Joy is yours to reclaim.

PRACTICE: CREATE YOUR OWN GROUND RULES

1. What will be your new guideposts on this journey? If it's helpful, make your own rules or touchstones about Joy. The world has handed you rules for far too long; it's time to make your own.
2. What do you believe about Joy? What do you know to be true?
3. You will know they are the right rules for you if you feel a whole body *Yes* when you read them, if they bring you a feeling of expansiveness or lightness. If they make you tense or contract, they may be a rule you have been given but do not believe.
4. Write them down, sing them in the shower, or record them and play them back to yourself in a headset; you will know when they feel right to you.
5. And if you don't want any rules, even of your own making, that's your freedom too. Maybe you want this journey to be open and see where it leads you. This is your road map to design.

PART II

RECLAIM YOUR TOOLS

CHAPTER 6

Ask, Don't Tell

WHY *NOT* ME?

After Steve and I received Zubin's diagnosis, we wanted to hit the Rewind button and say, *Let's try this again, for the love of whatever is holy in this world, please, give us a do-over.* Because now there was only one answer, and it wasn't the one we wanted.

And that's when the inevitable *Why?* started in our heads.

Why us?

Why this?

Why Zubin?

It's a familiar internal recording, from smaller daily pain points in life—when you get stuck in the worst traffic jam of all time—to my patients after they get a life-threatening diagnosis, and everything in between. *Why me?*

I repeated it incessantly through years of infertility. *Why me? Why my body?*

And that day, it rang ever so loudly. *Why us? Why Zubin?*

But after moments of painful stillness, the kind that make you want to scream but your chest is so incredibly tight you can't even breathe, one of us said, "*Why* not *us?*"

We, to this day, cannot quite remember which of us said it out loud in that traumatic space of time. But it was that first moment of feeling something in my body that I later recognized as my search for Justice in this unjust scenario. It just hung in the air with its own power, and we couldn't find a response.

Why not me? How do you answer that?

The only answers that arise try to desperately assert your worth as if hard things only happen to those who are undeserving, which is ludicrous even to write. Nothing happens to us because we are bad or not good enough.

The question alone, *Why me*, reveals our human arrogance. We recoil at the thought or reality of heart-piercing pain. We cannot and do not want to conceive of the fact that we could suffer.

Now, please hear me out, there is suffering you receive because of the fateful wheel of life and also that which is brought on us by those in power. As a Brown Sikh woman in America, I *know* that much of our suffering is unfair in the truest sense of that word. I wish oppression did not exist, and in the deepest interiors of my heart I fantasize about the ways the world could have played out differently so that was true. Life is beautiful and horrible; it is ugly, evil, and simultaneously triumphant. It is all that.

At the same time, you can exert your Chardi Kala—*Why not you* to pave a way through this adversity that is inclusive of Joy? When someone or a system has taken away some part of your power, do not, please, do not let them take yet one more thing. Let all the emotions be there, all the fear, the rage, the sadness; all are necessary. But do not let them take away the capacity to find your own Joy.

I get that this is hard. I get that you may need to stop here and take a pause. You may even feel annoyed with me. I, too, have felt such deep anger. And while Steve and I did have that moment of clarity—that moment of *Why not us?*—it wasn't always persistent in the beginning of this journey. In the first year after Zubin's diagnosis, we were visiting some dear friends with similarly aged children. No matter how hard I tried to just enjoy our kids playing together, I was spiraling deeper and deeper into thoughts of *Why me?* and *Why our family?* as I watched their easier life. At one point, my friend and I were talking about Zubin's diagnosis, and I retreated back to *Why us?* All I can remember is her answer.

Tanmeet, we are all vulnerable. It could be any of us.

I was so upset with these words, so hurt by what felt like an obtuse statement as she sat there with healthy children and no other discernible tragedy in her life. How dare she offer that as her response to me? Sure, we are all vulnerable, but she was still safe . . . and I was broken.

Her response was full of wise truth, but it was ill-timed. I was not ready to receive it.

Take a Pause

I acknowledge that my words may also not be coming at the right time for you. Please tend to your heart. Close this book. Take some deep breaths to expand your heart or make space. Scream, play loud music, or write out your anger. If you are able and there is green space around you, take a walk to breathe in the soothing scents of the trees around you. Or just choose a soothing word and repeat it over and over until it vibrates some ease into your heart. These actions may not clear the darkness instantly, but you can tend to yourself over and over in any challenging moment. And then come back when you feel ready.

There is no one side to life. If you love, if you live, you will hurt.

Many wisdom traditions teach this simple premise. In a timeless Buddhist story, a woman stricken with grief over the death of her firstborn child searches for someone who can bring her son back to life. She is taken to the Buddha who says he can help her if she brings him mustard seeds from a home where they have not experienced loss through death. She is unable to find such a home and returns humbled. As the Buddha explains, if you expect only happiness, you will be disappointed.

Each time you change the *Why me* story to *Why not me*, you soften resistance to the life in front of you. The one you're actually living, not the one you wished had played out. Asking insightful questions also feels bolder than just waiting for an answer. It is seeking Justice instead of waiting for it to be handed to you.

Take a Pause

If you are someone who has resisted Joy for far too long, and believe either you don't deserve it or you feel guilty experiencing moments of Joy when others do not, it is also a time to say out loud, *Why not me?* Why shouldn't you also be privy to Joy as part of the human experience? Just as we all have the vulnerability to suffer, we all have the birthright to feel Joy. Think about it as you get up each morning. What if, as you find fear and resistance coming your way, you think, *Why not me? Why not today? Why can't I be someone who also knows Joy?*

Amy Cuddy, highly acclaimed psychologist and TED speaker, studies the science behind the use of body language to change your mind. She says *expansiveness* (which I equate to a *Why not me* posture) *is not just an expression of power but then a cause of your power.* In her work, she shows that when people take on a more powerful, expansive pose for just two minutes, they may make changes in their biochemistry, such as a reduction in stress hormones, but most important, the pose affects behavior: You feel more confident, optimistic, and creative. People simply feel more powerful and in charge in these poses. This makes sense to me because there is evidence that individuals with power and status take up more space and marginalized individuals are expected to yield physical space to them. This has been my lived experience, but somehow seeing literature affirm this gives me less doubt that I am imagining the large white male in the airplane seat next to me who expects the armrest to be solely his while his legs also encroach on the small space I have left. Our body literally picks up nonverbal reminders constantly throughout the day—that I am smaller than that person, that they get more space than I do, and I can't push back.

At first, I received power poses as whitewashed woo, but now I see they are resistance in action. When oppression and chronic microaggressions are studied in communities, including in the form of bodily cues, these ways of learning to reclaim space are thought of, as Rae Johnson says, *embodied microresistances*. They become a way to push back and hold your ground in the face of the constant erosion of dignity that microaggressions create. In fact, these chronic bodily aggressions trigger your body's reactive nervous system and memories of the original oppression. Your body remembers its wounds but is also the fertile ground for their healing.

When life seems unfair, when you feel either subjugated by systems or the pain of your life's losses and tragedies, you feel smaller instead of larger. But when you reclaim emboldening physical stances, you can see your body as a source of personal and social power.

Why not you to now take up some space? Use this question to move your body into the space it is entitled to. The way you move your body can move your mind. Think about that. The way you make one simple shift with this question—*Why me?*—could shift how you physiologically and emotionally feel.

Take a Pause

Think of a challenge you are facing, small or large, right now in your life. And say to yourself, *Why not me?* out loud. Notice the difference in your body when you ask each question. When I say, *Why me?* I'm in a contracted, powerless shape. I play the victim.

When I say, *Why not me?* I stand in a place of power, straighter, chest out, legs apart and planted on the earth as if to say to this universe, *I hear you and, still, I stand up strong.* I imagine a lotus blooming out of the muddiest water and hear Maya Angelou's life-changing words, *Still I'll rise.*

I heard Amy Cuddy speak on a podcast about how these poses can make you more hopeful. She said something so powerful for me, how this hope can help you see other people not as predators, but as allies.... Standing big and wide can change how you see the world, as one that is more loving and kinder instead of one that is ready to take advantage of you. Remember that the ventral vagus, your soul connector to the world, is also stimulated by the way you see it. If you see the world as an ally, you can feel safer and calmer. To be clear: This doesn't mean you need to trust everyone or that harmful people don't exist. Rather, it is about trusting yourself to stand boldly in this world even if it has betrayed you yet again.

Although this question and body language shift your mind, this tool is not about *changing your thoughts*, as many self-help dictums prescribe. This is about *shifting the way you step into the world* so you can inhabit it differently and then take up the space you were meant to. This question is a powerful Justice move that shifts your body, mind, and heart toward more Joy.

You don't get to be Joyful by thinking you are different from anyone else. So, repeat *Why not me?* to yourself, over and over, until you see that you are human, you are vulnerable, and you are connected to the whole sea of humanity through this one undeniable truth. We will all feel unfathomable sadness. There is no way around it. We also all have the chance to feel our hearts soar, whether it's because of external systemic justice or personal triumph in our day-to-day lives.

Mark my words, Joy is and always has been with you all the way. It's time for you to rewrite this story.

WHY ARE YOU SO SAD?

You don't like being sad, do you?

I wanted to punch her, honestly. Instead, I think I just screamed something like *The FUCK I don't!* And in my head, thought, *Seriously, this is how she makes a living?*

I'll never forget that day. I had been crying so hard I couldn't see through the windshield as I drove. I knew I needed help, right then, and literally stopped the car to figure out how to safely drive forward. I hit the brakes and called Debbie.

I'm not even sure how to describe Debbie. If you look at her website, she's a licensed psychologist with a long career caring for both children and adults in crisis, and teaching on spirituality; she was also one of my then-new mentors in mind body medicine. So, you could say, people call Debbie when they need to find a way through their suffering.

I now know she is far bigger than any "About" page on a website could explain. She's my lifesaver in the truest sense. I wouldn't be the mother or teacher I am without her. I could dedicate this whole book to her because she's that big in my life, and if I go down a dark spiral of anxiety thinking about what to do when she dies, you'll find me crying in a corner.

But on this day, Debbie was still just a mentor who had offered to give me some guidance in this new shock-filled world of grief. She was someone I intuitively trusted, and for God's sake, I needed someone in that moment, so I gave in. I stopped the car and thought, *If I can't even fricking get through this car ride, what the hell am I going to do? And who the hell can help me?* Then, I remembered Debbie's offer: *Call me for a session and we can see how it goes.*

And that's the response I got. After crying so hard I could barely breathe, after telling her I was in desperate pain... *You don't like being sad, do you?*

But I have never forgotten that moment. It sank in, in such a heavy, visceral way, as my body held on to what my mind could not receive.

My questions to you in this book might make you angry. But stick with me please. Because what I can tell you is that the question Debbie asked shifted my journey and returned me to the one question that started my path to Joy. It brought me back to *Why not me?* Maybe that's too many questions right now, maybe you're confused. Just hang on.

Her question, even now when I remember that desperate drive, reminds me that I, like every other human on the face of this planet, will resist sadness or any challenging emotion like the plague. You, too, will try to squirrel your way out of it any way you possibly can. But I'm here to be your Debbie. I'm here to tell you, you don't like to feel uncomfortable and that's human. Facing your pain feels like danger.

But it's also a deeply human act to face pain and lovingly know it is yours to transform. And the real magic: Being aware of that pain and facing your discomfort in your body is a brave acceptance of yourself. If you can get comfortable in your own skin, you will reconnect with yourself in a way that can transform your life. If you want to get to your best life yet, you'll have to wade through some muddy shit.

But make no mistake. The act of running away from your emotions also creates deep mud, possibly the worst kind. When you suppress your emotions, brain imaging shows that you arouse your limbic system where powerful structures that process them sit, such as your amygdala (often referred to as the fear center). Trying not to feel sad or angry can make you feel more anxious or even rage filled. You think you're surviving by stuffing them down, that ignoring them puts a Band-Aid on them. But your body must manage them in the moment somehow.

Let that irony sink in. Trying not to feel...may hurt you the most.

The bigger injustice is that when your limbic system is aroused, your prefrontal cortex, the most evolved part of your brain that allows you to think with clarity and measure, is not able to function well. The cognitive energy it takes to distract you from your emotions only pushes that attention and energy into the primal recesses of your brain and hurts your ability to pay attention to the world around you.

And don't forget your ventral vagus nerve complex that innervates your facial structures and throat and helps you communicate to the world. How you move in the world may be off-kilter as this nerve *interoceptively* senses your discomfort. This is more impactful than you may realize. One study showed that by suppressing your emotions, you can even raise other people's blood pressure. As you rattle *your* nervous system, you may unsettle others around you as well.

I experienced this myself almost two decades ago when I was participating in a small group of nine people—all strangers at the time—learning mind body medicine skills. A few days in, after a powerful exercise, I revealed a deep sadness that I had yet to share with anyone other than my husband (we will get to that story later), one that I had thought I had suppressed quite skillfully. After I broke down, one of the group members said that they were so relieved to now see what was behind my *forced* smile. Others agreed that my *contrived* happiness made them feel uncomfortable. It wasn't until I came across this piece of neuroscience that I realized exactly what they meant. I was stuffing my sadness down to function in my life and hide a shameful truth. And in that action, others around me could feel a deep sense of *untruth* about me. What lay beneath the surface was much more visible than I had realized, and that veneer of false happiness had separated me from true connection all along.

Fortunately, there is a technique that neuroscience has shown can dampen this arousal while also allowing us to settle our limbic and nervous systems. This exercise can be a simple parallel practice to long-term therapy or deep inner work. Because, let's face it, you aren't always in a situation where you can discuss all your emotions, nor would you want to because you don't feel safe or simply need to get through the day. But if you can settle your body, you can think more clearly. It's called emotion labeling and it's as clear as it sounds. Label what you are feeling. No big nirvana like acceptance or reckoning, not the necessary cathartic and more difficult work of therapy, it's just simple calling out.

Matthew Lieberman, a neuroscientist at UCLA, has done some of the groundbreaking work on this technique, showing that despite people's predictions that labeling an emotion would make them feel worse, it does quite the opposite. And the specific noting dampens the limbic system while stimulating part of the prefrontal cortex. Participants feel more settled and clear thinking. I think of it as seeing the emotion within you instead of seeing it as all of you. *I am not sad, I am a person with a sad emotion.*

Take a Pause

If you're feeling a challenging emotion that is rattling your nervous system, take a few deep breaths and label it. *I am feeling sadness, fear, anxiety, anger,* whatever it may be. In a word or two, play *name that emotion*. The practice at the end of this section will give a way of doing this at more length, but for now just noticing is a small but powerful pause.

If a situation is challenging or seems unfair, you can acknowledge and label your emotions as a tool to settle your body and still stimulate your Joy practice. Last time I was at the cardiologist's office and we received more bad news about Zubin's heart failure, I said out loud to the doctor and my husband, *That news makes me so sad, and yet I know, in my core, that his heart has not failed him or me.*

I cannot change the effects of this devastating disease on my son's body and my family's life. But I can create a bigger and truer story than just the bad news given to me at any one time. That is Justice.

Along with the neuroscience, I have found in my own life and in caring for patients that bringing awareness to an emotion diminishes its power, even if sometimes just a bit, but enough to settle our systems more. It's energetically equivalent to looking someone in the eye and asserting your power. You aren't dismissing it; in fact, you are acknowledging it. You see the sadness, anger, or fear and it then lives more with you instead of holding as much power over you. Naming something gives you the power to work with it so you can take a stronger foothold in the world in that moment.

PRACTICE: EMOTION BUBBLES

Name what you feel. Get granular. Look it in the eye. Adopt curiosity as your approach. This is something you can do either at a set time in the day or as an on-the-spot mindfulness exercise.

1. Take a minute or two to sit quietly and start to focus on your breathing. Follow the rhythm of your breath and just notice what emotions may come into your awareness.
2. As you allow them to rise, imagine placing each emotion in a bubble and naming it. You could visualize blowing the bubbles away, watching them drift upward. Or even just watch them suspended in a bubble in front of you.
3. Realize how it is somewhat separate from you. It does not take you over. You are much more than that fear or anger or resentment.
4. As you see emotions as separate from you, you can see how dynamic they are. They are not as solid or unchanging as you

imagine them to be. They move in the air, they may get smaller or bigger in their bubbles, they may transform or melt into another emotion.

5. Just allow all of it to be there. It may be uncomfortable, but continually return to your breath for comfort and grounding and back again to the bubbles as you are able.

WHAT'S YOUR TRUTH?

This is hard to explain in regular words, so bear with me. The spirits were saying Zubin is a big-ass deal, kind of like a chairman of the board up there.

I wasn't sure I heard it right. And I didn't know whether to laugh or cry. Michael didn't exactly seem like the let-me-translate-the-spirits kind of guy. He was a dry wit, short-on-small-talk surgeon, the guy in medical school that I would have pegged for the cut-throat environment of the operating room right from the beginning. And here he was, on the phone, because he said he *had to talk* to me after visiting his shaman guide in Peru. How Michael even knew a shaman was beyond me, but at this point I was still grasping for any sign of meaning in my suffering. I was ready to take anything he gave me.

Turns out this man of few words not only visits a shaman, but this year he had also asked him to do a prayer for Zubin during one of their ceremonies.

That alone was touching and so unexpected. So, when he said we had to talk and then started it out like this, I was even more confused. But at this point, three years after Zubin's diagnosis, if there was one thing I had learned, it was to listen well. Look and listen for all signs of hope and Joy.

Okay, I'm with you, Michael, go on.

All right, it's like he's such a big deal that he doesn't even need to come down here to the human world. But he did because he wanted to work on some really big stuff. So, he picked a short life of big suffering because he didn't want to have to hang out here too long.

Okay, I'm not sure where this is going, I thought, but it seemed like a less traumatic explanation for Zubin's illness than his dystrophin gene accidentally skipping just one protein pair and then encoding so wrong that it caused catastrophe. Just a couple of letters reversed and now he won't walk, run, or live. No, I'll stick right now with this human-world-kind-of-sucks-and-he-wanted-a-quick-in-and-out explanation.

Okay, Michael, I'm with you, keep going.

I heard him take a big breath in before going on and thought, *Wow, not only have I never heard him talk for this long, but I think he's tearing up.*

All right, so when he came down here, he got to choose. Choose everything. How much suffering (a lot), how long he has to be here (not long), and who gets to come down with him.

Oh, so that's where this is going.

Now, I'm the one who needed a deep breath.

And he chose you and Steve and Sahaj and Neha. It was an honor that he chose you all. Because you knew that meant your soul would learn big lessons. All four of you were ready to go to the "next level" and Zubin was going to take you there.

Silence.

Neither of us said a word for what felt like a long time.

Deep breaths.

Zubin is here to teach me.

In the spirit of legendary thinker, Holocaust survivor, and psychiatrist Viktor Frankl's words, *Suffering without meaning is just that, suffering.* Your deep well of meaning is the same well that holds your pain and love. It's that important.

Find your belief system, the one that works for you. I offer you mine as an example, not because it is *the* truth but because it is my truth:

All that happens in my life, even the most painful parts, can have meaning and purpose for my soul's growth, purpose that I design. That a divine force, this universe, whatever you want to call it, something more vast, is always there for me, even when it doesn't appear that way. Not ever that it happens for a reason as others say. But everything that happens to me can have larger than myself purpose if I choose to meet it. I never deserve pain, but I sure as hell deserve to find meaning and Joy, no matter what.

The truth is that I have my religion and I also have my universal truth. They don't conflict with each other. So, what will be your truth? As long as it feeds your soul and doesn't impact others' safety and health, let it be your religion, your witchery, or even sheer luck, but let it be yours.

It really doesn't matter to me if you believe my truth; that's the beauty, it gets to be mine and be right. My truth doesn't mean I don't get sad, angry, or worried. But eventually, I also trust that those emotions will deepen my relationship with Joy in a way I cannot see at that moment. When I honor their worth, I trust *myself* more deeply. My body knows what it's doing.

Take a Pause

What if you realize that each time you wrestle with something difficult, you get closer to your truth? That all you encounter can be a bigger teacher for you than even the solution to solve it. In the same way your body gives you signals to move your hand from a hot stove, your mind and body send you emotional cues to protect you from more pain. Your sadness can give you the message of what you really love. Your outrage is a sign of how much you care in this world. Remember even in the dark times, you can hold to your *deeper why* or your own *ground rules* to lead you back to your truth. You and only you get to decide how and when you will move through the darkness, but Justice is holding on to the belief that you can. You didn't ask for this pain; you definitely don't deserve it. But you never need to earn your right to move through it with Joy at your side.

Everything that happens to me deserves my filter of Justice: *What do I deserve to receive even when I didn't deserve* this? The truth is that when you are remapping the carved grooves of your brain to find the meaning in suffering, you change your perspective from one of sufferer to a seeker of beauty. Not because the world necessarily did right by you, but *you can do right by you*, regardless.

Five years ago, I broke my foot in two places in the silliest mishap and I went through all the expected funk that comes with being limited by a knee scooter and then a walking boot and still feeling the pain over six months later. As someone for whom a daily walk is a deep salve, I wondered—angrily, I'll admit—*What gifts will I possibly find in this?* Seeing life from Zubin's perspective was an obvious one, but there was an even bigger one.

Something I could never have predicted happened. When I broke my foot, it put a stress on my household that we had not experienced before. I couldn't lift, move, or do any personal care for Zubin. And we realized what a fragile thread our family hung on when one of the two primary caregivers was now not able to do her role. My then fourteen-year-old son offered to be a helper. *Why can't I lift and care for Zubin,* he proposed.

We were desperate for some way to navigate this new obstacle. So, Sahaj stepped up. He lifted. He transferred. He did personal care. I get teary eyed even writing about it because the level of compassion I saw in him was heart opening. I don't know how many fourteen-year-olds could use a handheld urinal on their thirteen-year-old brother without flinching. Over and over, he was our strongest (literally) asset.

And so even after I got strong enough again, Sahaj now is part of our caring force, more capable and trustworthy than any caregiver I could find. And beyond how he has helped our family, I may never know how this deepening of his experience with his brother may have changed the fabric of who he is and what he will give to this world. I see this same compassion in my youngest child who has just started at the same school as Zubin. On her own, Neha seeks him out, advocating when he cannot, and reporting on his safety and successes. *Zubin if you chose these two, you chose well.* Gifts are everywhere . . . if you look for them.

Take a Pause

If you're up most nights still wondering *Why me*, realize you may be at the precipice of *your* truth. You don't need to stop feeling sad, frustrated, or angry. Nurture those emotions. Get curious. And keep asking. Keep screaming. You may eventually scream your way into *Why not me*, and then your truth, and it doesn't matter how long that takes. Slowly but surely, the screaming will metamorphose into sheer marvel. And when the ratio of marvel to anger tips enough, you will have walked into a different kind of bliss.

PRACTICE: WHAT IS YOUR TRUTH?

This may be the most challenging question in the book. And I wish there were an easy exercise for it. The truth is that asking the question is the way to find your answer. But let's get you "warmed up" as we would for any new physical challenge.

1. Take out your journal or voice app or do this in movement or meditation. Think of a challenge in your life. Don't start with the hardest ones. Write, speak, or muse on what that challenge was/is. Give it a small story, just a few sentences at the most, to get it into your psyche for the moment.

2. Then, write what you think was *your* meaning in that challenge. How do you make sense of how that impacted you for your own highest way of being in the world? What did it teach or offer you in your life, if anything?
3. This will be the most challenging when it comes to the evil and oppression we have referred to. In those cases, you can try thinking not of what that gave you, but instead what you can now give to yourself or the world after surviving it. And you might need more space or time from the experience to do this exercise—that's your call.
4. Give this part, the sense, the meaning, a wider story. More writing, talking, or musing. It deserves more space than the pain took up, so reclaim that.
5. Do this with challenges until you start to see connecting threads of truth emerge for yourself. Compile that truth somewhere you can see, hear, or feel it over and over. It can also change with time, just like you. Think of it as a narrative of your life that deserves your attention often.
6. Also, your truth may just come to you quickly without this reviewing of your challenges. You will know because when you say it, you will feel a whole body *Yes*, a lightness or release. Listen to that. Your body knows.

CHAPTER 7

Don't Just Accept Everything

TURN TOWARD IT

It was December 2008, a little over one year from the fateful Monday, and Zubin and I flew to Corpus Christi. I had heard of a podiatrist there who had designed a machine using his own form of micro electrical stimulation along Chinese meridians to treat chronic pain syndromes. A family of a young boy with DMD explored this treatment; that boy was now still able to walk at an age when the natural history of the condition predicted otherwise. The news spread like wildfire in the DMD community. Even as an Integrative Medicine physician, I didn't completely grasp his hypothesis of how this worked. But I knew it was unlikely to be harmful and that's all this desperate mama needed to spend a lonely Christmas week with Zubin in Texas.

Lonely is how it felt without Steve who could not get vacation time. And with Zubin who still had significant speech challenges and was far from being able to have a back-and-forth dialogue with me. We stayed at a condo on a long road out of town toward the water on a recommendation from another family who had come to do this treatment. They said at least going back to the beach was a retreat for them in the middle of what was otherwise a grueling week. But with no conversation and bleak winter weather, those four daily rides back and forth for treatments were tortuous, long, and desolate. I kid you not when I say I spent the entire drive, both ways, crying. Nonstop. In fact, I cried most of the week. At the clinic, on the drive, getting myself and Zubin ready in the morning, all day, all night. It felt like I was stuck in a movie, a cross between the two of us on long roads in *Thelma and Louise* (although with far less laughter) and the desperate search of *Lorenzo's Oil*.

But there was something radical about this aloneness, to acknowledge my spiritual desolation without anyone else there to resolve it. There was nowhere to hide the tears and no one to hide them from. For the first few days, Zubin just watched me cry with an indiscernible look of either contentment or obliviousness. We would go to the clinic in the morning, back in the evening, and then I would do a treatment on him at night. Just the two of us, Zubin laying there with the sticky pads and electrodes on his legs and arms, an alien-like device at his feet making beeps intermittently, and the silence of my aching heart.

Four days in, we were in the clinic getting one of our daily treatments while Zubin watched a movie. I was crying, as usual, and he looked up from the screen and smiled at me in a different way. I couldn't quite put my finger on it, and then he went back to watching the movie. When we checked out of the clinic that day, the woman at the front desk was giving me more instructions and, yes, I cried through that all. Zubin stood at my side and spontaneously embraced my legs. He had never done this before. I looked down at him as he squeezed, and he said, as clear as anything, *I love you, Mama.* I cried even harder. Not only had he strung a full sentence together, but he had never said these words, ever. For the rest of that week, he said it several times a day.

There was something mystical about that trip. We were alone on a quest. And maybe he could feel not only my love but also my unmasked pain. Maybe he could feel my involuntary softening to my grief, the floodgates open after a year of full-on resistance to this life. And maybe I opened his heart in a way as well. Either way, it changed our relationship permanently. To this day, he tells me *I love you* many times a day, spontaneously.

You don't need to have a solo quest for a cure to feel your pain. What I had was the experience of letting myself be sad and allowing it to flow uninterrupted. It was cathartic and wildly painful, but something broke open inside me. Now where there was only darkness in my heart, there was also some space for ease. Was it acceptance? Not quite. But it was definitely a turning toward the pain.

S = P × R

Not every instance of turning toward your pain must be as dramatic as that feature film–like story. When I was crying in Corpus Christi nonstop, the magic was that I just let it happen. And when you stop resisting, your body literally softens, to yourself. True liberation in your body is initiated by not only your desire but by your nurturing self-love connecting you to who you really are in any one moment. That is how you gift yourself Justice when the world seems to have none to give.

In my TEDx Talk, I spoke of a simple equation I learned that clarifies how important this is and utterly changed my journey.

$S = P \times R$

Suffering equals pain times resistance.

There is pain in this life, the P in the equation. We all have it. But you may have heard that suffering is optional. I would say yes and no. If you have pain, you will suffer, for varying amounts of time. But at some point, *how much* may be modifiable.

When you continually resist the pain, try to push it away and wish you didn't have it, then you have amplified suffering. Remember how I didn't want to be sad? That was my R, my resistance. And it multiplied my suffering.

But when you allow the sadness to be there, your resistance is zero and then there is no suffering.

Just the pain. And then we can get down to business and work with that.

Take a Pause

It can be challenging to get honest with yourself on this one. Where are you resisting and causing more suffering? Where can you gently soften to what is happening? That can be as simple as saying out loud that it is, in fact, happening. Because usually we create a dialogue in our head about how we wish it were not. It doesn't mean you love, accept, or even forgive it. You just acknowledge the truth. It is happening.

STOP THE FIXING

One of the reasons you feel so much pain is that you want the source of the pain to be gone. This is natural, whether it is physical injury, loss, or suffering imposed by another. There's nothing wrong with wanting it gone, but in most cases, this may not be realistic. And even when it is, you need sharp clarity on your next best action, which, remember, requires settling your nervous system first.

Recently, Steve had been suffering from debilitating shoulder pain, the kind that keeps you up at night and has you screeching in agony after simply reaching the wrong way. As most physical pain does, it was making him irritable and frustrated. On a walk, we talked about how hard it is to feel the physical agony. But then he revealed that every time he feels the pain, he also feels fear for the future, that he won't be able to lift or transfer Zubin. He admitted this deep fear of not being a useful caregiver, that he is only getting older and maybe this pain will be a chronic challenge.

His fears are all valid. But they're not happening *right now.* Only the pain is. I asked him what would be left if there was nothing to fix right now in this moment. After he huffed a bit (I know, none of these questions are easy!), his body eased, his shoulders softened, and he admitted, it was then just the pain. Not all the future anxiety. Just the pain itself. Then, he was able to get clarity that he needed to get more medical help, adhere better to a stretching program, take anti-inflammatory supplements and medication, and so on. He was able to see more clearly through the overwhelm, the layers he had himself added on.

Take a Pause

It can be an overwhelming task to attain even a small bit of calm when pain, whether emotional or physical, is present in the here and now. But that might mean it's time to ask a question instead of looking for the solution alone. Imagine a present challenge, if there was *nothing to fix* in this moment—no pain to resolve, no grief to end, no system to fight, no boss to contend with—if there was nothing to fix, what would be left? Are you layering suffering on top of the pain, making it harder and more complicated to contend with? No blame or self-judgment here; just have curiosity. What is left? Can you see it with a bit more clarity?

Steve's shoulder pain is an everyday example but important all the same. There is also catastrophic loss. My friend lost her young husband unexpectedly last year, a devastating shift in her life. If she asks this question, *What if there was nothing to fix?* she might just see deep soul sadness. And that is brutal. But it is sadness that is not compounded further by any regrets of the relationship in the past or the future fear of a life that will never be Joyful again. This kind of sadness eventually can be softened or transformed so that she can have the capacity to feel other emotions alongside it. The more we layer on our own fear, the more our mind and body spiral into future anxieties. When that happens, the more rigid and untenable our thought patterns become. We become stuck in the pile on.

Take a Pause

That pile on is all the stories you tell yourself about the present challenge. If you are angry that you are suffering, it is easy to spin narratives—why it's frustrating to feel angry yet again, how this feels like it will never get easier—but seeing the emotion alone can even make a potential benefit of anger, such as motivation, more accessible. Remember that seeing and validating your emotions allows you to regulate your nervous system with more ease and power. It's then a single emotion, not your entire story. You are far bigger than that.

THE SECRET

Ed held the talking stone longer in silence than he ever had. As he rubbed the calming divot on its underside and looked down, the group felt the heaviness of what sat within him.

Ed was an army veteran, now here in my small group to learn practices to find *peace and Joy* again, he said. He had shared with us already in the first four groups how he had been deployed to Afghanistan, in his words, *somehow survived*, and now was home with his wife and ten-year-old son. He thought simply being home with them would lead to more Joy again. But now that he had returned, he felt daily tension and conflict in his marriage and he found himself growing impatient with his son, yelling more than he wanted to admit. He had yet to feel the peace he had imagined and that angered him even more, he had revealed.

Today when the stone was passed to him, he lingered silently. And when he raised his gaze, his eyes were wet.

I've been so upset about my anger that I've created even more of the exact thing I want to squash.

He pushed his thumb down into the depression on the back of the stone. And then took a deep breath.

It's not my fault that my job, the way I got paid, for so long, was to be angry and fight. And now I'm just supposed to turn that off? Like it's a switch?

His voice quickened and got louder.

I'm a goddamn human being, not a light switch.

He looked around the circle now, slowly. And then slowed his voice as well.

I've spent so much time thinking my irritability and anger were my fault but now I realize that they are just part of me. Just a part. They seem smaller now and I'm bigger than that.

He smiled slowly. *I'm bigger than that.*

And he lightly passed the stone.

What you hear often is that acceptance of *what is* will bring you peace and even Joy, eventually. That if you stay in the present moment, you will finally get to bliss. I won't discount the power of that wisdom, but let me explain a nuance I have found to be even more true.

Turning toward the present moment, the pain, the hard emotions, whatever is in front of you, is not only the way to get to Joy. It actually *is* the Joy, right there and then. Every time you turn toward your life as it unfolds in front of you—and, more important, see your full self as you unfold into your life—you settle your resistant and rattled nervous system that may be stuck in past regret or future anxiety. You tell yourself you are safe. These emotions are okay, they are part of being human. You move into your frontal cortex where you have clarity and a sharper mind. You open your chest and heart. You inhabit a power pose.

The Joy is feeling it all... the anger, the rage, the frustration, the sadness... and learning you don't have to be overwhelmed by it. In fact, the more you can see and name exactly the emotion you are feeling, while deeply knowing it's okay to feel it, the more you can see yourself as vast as the sky above you and your emotions as clouds, some large or dark and some billowy and small. You can hold them all without being defined completely by any single one of them.

This is the Joy of being fully alive.

CHAPTER 8

Your Love Matters

WHO YOU LOVE MATTERS

Angela's tears flowed freely as she recalled the horror of the first aid helicopters that arrived with men throwing out toilet paper, an insulting and inadequate Band-Aid to the suffering people below. She cried about the condescending words from President Trump and his administration and expressed shame in being treated like *animals.*

In the fall of 2017, Hurricane Maria struck the island of Puerto Rico, testing not only its geographic resilience but the capacity of its inhabitants to weather some of their most devastating losses yet. Lives, homes, businesses, all washed out in the wake of a disaster so big that recovery is still taking place today. To add to the suffering, the United States government would act too slowly and callously, with a level of response that had no match for the destruction. The losses lingered heavily when I visited in May 2019 as part of an effort to share mind body medicine skills with social workers, health-care professionals, and teachers. One hundred fifty participants from across the islands of Puerto Rico attended to help heal the toll of the emotional devastation in their communities.

Angela, one of the social workers, told me she had dismissed her own trauma because it wasn't *as bad* as that of others she knew. Her emotions felt *weak* and *childish* because *there was too much work to do* and she needed to be *strong enough* to do it. Her anger and grief were palpable as she described what and who she had lost as a single mother, sister, and daughter, and all she had seen taken away from her community.

After exercises in self-compassion, she saw that her emotions were not only *okay* but necessary. And that instead of wanting to be *strong for others*, she knew she needed first to learn to accept herself so that she could step fully into the work of reclaiming Justice for her people. She had experienced, for the first time, an understanding that her anger and sadness were not limiting failures for her work but powerful fuel for it. And not just parts of her to accept, but most important, to love.

If you love yourself, you step toward your own Justice.

This is science-based truth that is accessible to all of us. Self-compassion isn't some touchy-feely BS or a tool only for people who have money and time, it is a direct path to Joy. You can love yourself because you deserve it, plain and simple.

I spoke with Angela recently and she says she still works on this daily. After committing to the first step of recognizing her own inner critical voice, she realized a bigger truth: *Just because I felt a lack of love or care from others, in the aftermath of that suffering, did not mean I could not give myself what I needed most.*

Loving yourself is hard work, and frankly the phrase is nebulous and sometimes overwhelming. We will lay out some steps to start, and as always, you will pave your own right path. Yes, it is hard work—trust me, I have to practice it daily—and it usually feels worse before it feels better. So, I don't promise loving yourself is an instant path to a rainbow moment of bliss.

But compassion has a secret superpower worth knowing. It supports that vagal pathway of safety so that as you experience your pain or the pain of another, you inhibit your defense pathways. You work on compassion for yourself and others, not just to feel better or give love, but to feel safer. It is a golden-lit sling to carry you through this world.

What the world doesn't give you is inexcusable.

But what you can give yourself is Justice.

YOUR BRAIN KNOWS THE DIFFERENCE

When you berate yourself, your brain and body feel attacked and look for comfort. Anyone who has been an adolescent or parents one will understand this well. If you want a teen to change a habit and use criticism in directing how they should change—*Why can't you learn?*—most likely they will repeat that habit. Harsh words signal your midbrain centers to be fearful, feel unsafe, and put you into fight-or-flight mode. Your brain then looks for ways to just survive; thriving and growing do not fit into the plan in that moment. Instead, your brain often looks for comfort in the exact thing you are trying to change, the habitual patterns that usually do not serve you: escaping the pain through overspending, scrolling your phone, using substances, or more. Whether you are speaking harshly to yourself or someone else is, your brain sees it the same way, as an attack to fear and flee. And take out the neuroscience for a moment; berating yourself is also simply an awful experience, a moment of suffering.

Researchers show through sophisticated brain imaging that when you activate these midbrain fear centers, you put a brake on taking action. It's as if your brain is saying, *Slow down, it's not safe out there in the world.* You feel almost imprisoned in your mind and lose motivation to make change, in yourself or the world. The implications are that internal self-criticism can be an extension of external threat in the body. And that self-compassion can then be a way to activate safety from within. In fact, when you extend compassion to yourself, you see that it is possible to reduce the fight-or-flight stress response as evidenced in less reactivity in both your cardiovascular system and emotional centers of your brain. Hear this well: self-compassion settles your heart and body.

I think of this science when I recall all the ways I have been taught that my responses to the injustices of the world are wrong. I clearly remember one of my supervisors sitting me down and offering his unsolicited, punitive feedback about my advocacy in meetings: *You are too angry, too negative.* What if, instead, he had reassured me that my emotions are human and reasonable? Would I have felt a bit more sure-footed in this world that had made me so angry?

Studies also show that using this tool puts you in a state in which you are more conscious of your choices and have more clarity. You can operate out of your prefrontal cortex where you have the capacity to make decisions and feel motivated. Even when the world is not compassionate toward you, you can use the Justice of self-compassion to make it safer for you to step into it.

YOU WILL HAVE TRIPSTER DAYS

One night at dinner, my daughter, in second grade at the time, told us about her school day. Amid a long, winding story (she can masterfully spin stories like no other!), Neha mentioned that she had tripped on her jacket while running across the playground. The jacket was tied around her waist and one of the sleeves was a bit too long so, in her excitement, she had tripped over it, right onto the asphalt.

I admit my first parental instinct was to remind her to tie her jacket tighter.

Thankfully, before I could berate her, she went on, *It was so embarrassing. . . . I'm so stupid.*

Embarrassment was a reasonably human response, an uncomfortable feeling, but her self-condemnation was the suffering she quickly laid on top. So young, trusting of so many things, but not of herself.

I held back and saw how admonishing her would have only compounded her self-image of incompetence.

Instead I offered, *Sometimes, it's just a tripster day. . . .*

And she laughed in a way that made me tear up. Because in that moment, she saw her human-ness; she saw that *slipping up* is universal and that *a tripster day* just happens.

We aren't stupid.

We aren't self-sabotaging.

We're just like a second grader, so excited to get to the playground.

And sometimes we trip.

PRACTICE: NOTICING YOUR SELF-TALK

Being aware of the way you speak to yourself is a critical first step in cultivating self-compassion.

1. Think of the last time you made a mistake, small or large. Remember, without judgment, what you said to yourself. Or notice from here on how you speak in these situations.
2. What are the words you use? Would you say these words to a good friend in the same situation? Notice how many times you say *I should*... how many times you say you aren't good enough... how many times someone does it *better than me*. Just stop and notice. For some, writing down these words can be an eye-opener. For others, it may be too painful. For now, just notice in any way that works for you.
3. What are the words you would use with a friend in the same situation? Write those down or say them out loud and notice what you feel in your body when you read or hear these. They may feel different in your body than your own internal speak.

SUPERHUMAN

Zubin's bones are now so paper-thin from chronic steroids that a fracture can happen with even simple movements. One night while Steve was stretching Zubin's legs in his nightly routine to prevent early contractures, he turned him in a way that caused a break in his femur.

Zubin never stood up again on his own two legs.

No forgiveness from myself or Zubin could ease Steve's conscience. He was beyond regretful and blamed himself repeatedly. One night, I asked Steve how he was ever going to get past this. It didn't matter for me to sadly remind him that Zubin's last days on his feet were nearing, no matter what happened that night.

Me: *You're human, Love, you made a mistake.*

Steve, without hesitation: *There wasn't room for error in this situation.*

Me: *Oh, I didn't realize that you're superhuman.*

You strive to do your best, but you also must accept where you fall at any given time.

That is the superhuman power in all this.

If you're asking yourself, *How do I accept myself when I regret an action and know I need to improve?* Ah, that's where the magic is. Think about it; that is not inconsistent at all with self-compassion. You want to improve exactly *because of* your love for yourself, because you care and want better. It's why parents want their kids to get enough sleep or eat nourishing foods, because they care for them. Self-compassion is at the root of all desire to change.

Take a Pause

If you are actively trying to change or make a new habit, love needs to be one of your main tools. And nowhere in any dictionary have I seen a definition of accountability that includes shame. That is our pile on. *No one attempt defines your larger capacity for change, only your human-ness at trying.*

My patients are often scared to tell me they weren't successful with change.

Patient: *I didn't want to come tell you I slipped up.*

. . . Deep pause of fear, often with a downward gaze . . .

Me: *It's a slippery world.*

We plan, we hope, we try. And yet, we make mistakes, we fall short, we disappoint ourselves.

Welcome to the human race.

It's hard out there.

To make change. To accept our emotions. To feel loss and grief. To muster hope.

It's all hard.

And it's so slippery.

Get up and try again. And remind yourself there are billions of other humans getting back up and trying every day. You're not superhuman or any different.

Self-compassion has a continuum of difficulty, there's no doubt, and some days, the practice is easier than others. But the important part is to keep practicing. The more you can accept and love yourself in any moment, no matter what you are striving for—or even failing at—the more likely your brain and body will be on your side. The more likely you will feel safe enough to go forward in the journey.

Take a Pause

When you accept your own imperfections, it also makes it easier to see others' flaws and think, *I've been there* or *I get that*. That's the ventral vagus nerve kicking in, making us connect even stronger to others, but most important, to ourselves. Kristin Neff, one of the pioneering researchers in self-compassion, says this principle of common humanity is one of the core components of this work.

PRACTICE: LOVINGKINDNESS AS SELF-TALK

After you notice how you speak to yourself, try to make space for other words as well. I add a lot of *So silly* to myself, making the mistake playful like the *tripster day*. This may be the most challenging part of the practice. At least for me, it is. My default is criticism. But often practicing lovingkindness can be a way to flex this self-compassion muscle and send kinder words your way. Try placing a picture of yourself as a child out where you can see it every day. I have one framed in my office to remind myself to be gentle. Traditionally, lovingkindness meditation is practiced first as a blessing for yourself before sending it outward to others. Let's use that suggestion.

1. The practice is to, as usual, notice your breath first for a few minutes so you can downregulate your nervous system. I like to then breathe into my heart a few times, expanding it with the inhale and sending out love with the exhale.
2. You will then use phrases as your anchor just as you have done with the breath. You repeat the phrases and if (and when) your mind wanders, return your attention to the phrases.
3. You can take the liberty of making the phrases yourself so the following are just suggestions. The sweet spot seems to

be three or four phrases repeated over and over so that they become a touchstone in the meditation, like your breath. If your mind strays or you feel silly, remember you can just keep coming back to the phrases as your anchor.

4. Some suggestions: *May I be healthy, May I be safe, May I have Joy, May I live with ease.* But make them your own. *May I have calm, May I have peace, May I know love.* Whatever feels right to you.
5. Start by taking a few deep breaths to come into your body. Eyes open or closed, whatever feels safest, and then repeat the phrases, all three or four, one time, and then again several times as a set.
6. Do this daily if able or a few times a week. In one to two months, do the practice of noticing your self-talk again. Has it changed or softened at all? Remember, this is a process.

SAFETY AT YOUR FINGERTIPS

Tanmeet, where are you?

That question on the phone call I had just received was simple, yet shocking. *Where are you?* I had somehow scrambled my calendar and thought I had the morning off, but I was scheduled to be in clinic to teach the residents. I had never made such a big blunder in my schedule. And now the residents were waiting and getting late, themselves. And that's when my barrage of negative words started, instantly. I had to stop the car because my inner critical voice was too disruptive to concentrate on driving.

How could you do that? How could you be so stupid? Idiot, careless, irresponsible... I heard all of it in my mind. And loudly. And no amount of *Remember to accept yourself, extend self-compassion* reminders were coming in to soften it.

I stopped the car, intuitively placed a hand on my heart—I think because it felt so damn bad to berate myself—and took a few breaths. I could feel my nervous system softening. And then I was able to hold two things to be true: I could be curious about my self-talk while not accepting it as absolute truths about myself. I learned something critical in that moment. That this act of touch could be the best first thing for me to do no matter what. Self-compassion is hard work, but physical touch can uplevel this Justice tool in your favor.

Humans are wired for touch. It is how you comfort a baby or a friend. It is your first instinct when a loved one shares their grief, to hug them or hold their hand. And when you hear the inner voice of your mind, do for yourself what humans need most. Reassure yourself that you are loved, that you are safe, in this moment. You can hug yourself if you like. I am usually in a space where a light touch, such as a finger or hand on my heart, feels more inconspicuous, but you do you. I invite you to see how this feels when you are practicing self-compassion, no matter what kind of internal speak has begun. Many times, the more primal language of touch can shift your heart to compassion more quickly than words.

The science of touch supports this invitation. Safe touch, from others or yourself, promotes the secretion of oxytocin, soothes you, and makes you want to connect to others. Functional MRI (fMRI) studies show, when patients anticipate threat or stress, the areas of the brain that light up are *turned off* when they are touched by a partner. Let me say that again. Safe touch turns off threat. You can give yourself a piece of calm and Justice in any moment by turning off the threat of self-criticism.

And remember this very important piece. The critical voice doesn't always go completely away; in fact, it rarely does. The Justice is not in completely extinguishing it, but instead in finding a different way of relating to it that allows you to always be growing into your best self. It is exactly this path of responding differently to yourself that will carve new pathways in your brain and heart to Joy.

PRACTICE: MOVING ASIDE

If touch doesn't work or feel right in that moment, you can try to literally *step* out of your thoughts. Let's say you just heard your own thoughts about what a failure you are. You've noticed them, maybe even without judgment. You may have even reframed or tried touch but you need more. Take a deep breath to signal to yourself that you are creating some space and step to the side. Yes, actually step, roll, or gesture to the side, whatever is available to your body. Sometimes, I even plié, ballet style, or stomp. Make your step your own. As if you are moving to the side of your thoughts. You are now in new space, on fresh ground. It's a new moment. Try again.

LOVE MATTERS. PERIOD.

I didn't know Claire more than as a good friend of one of my coworkers. Until she had her first child. Then, I heard her name even more often. On that night, she had to deliver the baby alone. Claire's partner developed a severe headache in the middle of her labor and the physicians in the emergency room discovered a massive tumor in his brain. One that would need urgent treatment and take his life over the course of that next short year.

I thought often that year about the ways I had no idea what Claire was going through. And I thought about all the ways I yet wanted to try to imagine the pain. The pain of loss, grief, rage, and anger. The pain of the sweet first year of your child being overtaken by a loss so large. I felt an inexplicable desire to reach out and wrote her a letter that asked for no reply. I remember saying on those pages that even though I could never *know* her pain, I did feel pain in my heart *with her* and I knew how difficult it was to suffer. And that none of us deserves to suffer alone, without knowing how much their story has touched even a complete stranger. I sent her compassion not because she necessarily needed mine but because we are all human and need each other.

A few years later, I did meet Claire.

I'm Tanmeet. I know we don't know each other. . . .

And before I could finish, she hugged me tightly, both of us teary-eyed.

Your letter was one of the most soothing things I received in that painful time.

Someone saw me, she said, *and was holding me, even from afar. I wasn't alone.*

A stranger's words on a piece of paper, but a piece of Justice to her all the same.

Compassion has that power. It says to someone, *I feel with you*. Because in so many ways, I am you. I am human. I hurt, I grieve, I love, and *even though I cannot ever know your pain, I am willing to step into it with you*.

When you feel and accept your own pain more deeply, you feel the pain of the world as well. It's not an onerous thing—although I won't lie, it can be tiring. But only in the way that love can move through us so strongly and carve deep, weighty rivers. Because when you love yourself, you are better able to love all the Claires of the world you don't know.

PRACTICE: SELF-COMPASSION

Let's review the work once more. Remember this is work that starts to *work on you* after a while. The effort is worthwhile.

1. Notice the mess. It's a human mess, we all have it. How do you talk to yourself?
2. Start accepting it as part of you, part of being human and imperfect.
3. Find other words and often. Find words that feel authentic but allow space for your human-ness. Can you find words that still feel true but are more loving?
4. Use touch as needed for safety or when language is not feeling easy. A finger or hand on the heart, a self-hug. Give yourself nurturing care for this hard work.

5. Put up a childhood picture of yourself in your home or work desk. Look at that version of yourself often and practice speaking to them the way you want to speak in your mind. If you love writing, write letters to that child to encourage them.
6. And try to imagine or literally, physically, in any way that is available to you, moving apart from your thoughts as needed to create space for new ways of speaking to yourself.
7. Rinse and repeat all day because that's what we do. Remember the goal is not having the language go away completely but creating a new way of relating to it.

CHAPTER 9

Your Body Is Your Home: Settle In

THE WHOLE ENVELOPE

Early in my Integrative Medicine training a mentor told me, *Tanmeet, when you are with a patient, remember to listen with the whole envelope of your skin.*

I admit, I was confused. But now, I've come to understand why your body is your most powerful tool for presence and listening to others, and most important, to yourself. Your body is an ever-present anchor in this moment. And because it is always here and listening, it contains all your memories, pain, *and* your capacity for Joy.

Being in your whole envelope, an *embodied* approach, can develop with exercises that put you squarely into your body instead of disconnecting from it. My mentor was referring to mindful listening as one way. But you can also do this through movement, breath, connection, and expression like writing or art. In fact, your nervous system has specialized neurons that sense your body in space and allow you to *balance and orient* by intaking sensory data and then using this as information for your next movement, a process termed *proprioception*, from the Latin roots *proprius* for "one's own" and *capere*, "to grasp." I think of it as your body's own unique grasp on receiving the world.

Take a Pause

Let this sink in for a moment. Your nervous system has specialized receptors to sense *where your body is and how it moves forward.*

And remember that while your body is receiving the world, your brain is scanning your inner landscape for messages as remembered signals.

A tightness in the chest—*This person is not safe.*

A fluttering in the gut—*I don't feel good about doing this.*

That's your *interoceptive awareness* we've discussed, your Spidey senses. The more you arrive into your body's envelope—the practices in this section are only a few ways—the more it becomes a powerful sensory tool. It is in your *body* that you can untangle oppressive stories your *mind* has held on to. Untangle is different than dismiss. You are not negating the reality of your pain, merely loosening its tight grip on your body.

We talked about the power of safe touch in self-compassion work. In that context, it literally is a vehicle to meet yourself *lovingly and safely* in your body. Touch also can be a way to remember to *feel into* your body. When you hug someone (whom you want to touch), debatably somewhere between six and twenty seconds, you produce oxytocin and decrease cortisol, and your body relaxes. Your blood pressure and heart rate both decrease, and you feel safe. Instead of focusing on how long the hug should be, I focus on sensing when my body finally surrenders into relaxation in a hug to know that it's working. In other words, I can *listen to my body* to know its truth. Even the touch of warm temperature to your body can be a soothing companion, literally increasing your personal warmth and ability to trust. The brain senses this warmth as a safety signal.

Take a Pause

There are entire bodies of work on this skill of interoception, urging you to use it to *locate* your emotions as well. When you feel an emotion, consider trying to locate it and just have awareness of it there in physical form—*I feel that anger as a fire in my gut, I feel that sadness in my throat as a tightening*. That awareness alone is liberation because you are literally settling into your own skin. Being true to your own feeling experience is a way to be true to yourself.

In Part 1, I spoke of the circle of communication between the different parts of your nervous system. If you attend to this cross-talk, as I would call it, it is a way to enter your body's envelope more deeply. You can hone this skill through mindful observation of your sensations or locating your emotions to fine-tune your awareness.

There are so many ways to enter your body, over and over. The essence to understand here is that your body can learn how to listen. Researchers have studied yoga practitioners and meditators to show that you can improve this sense of interoceptive awareness over time. And that is how you create new neural pathways, new grooves of Joy in your body's awareness. When you enter your own envelope, you become a coconspirator of your life with your body that calls to you often.

Important note: If you have experienced a great deal of trauma, working with a skilled trauma/somatic therapist who can help you establish a context of safety in your body is a critical step in this path.

PRACTICE: HONING YOUR BODY AWARENESS

The key to hone your interoceptive awareness is to practice *noticing* without getting swept up in your mind's stories.

For this exercise, let's use your body itself. Pair a regular activity in the day with a chance to *check in* with your body. Maybe it's washing the dishes, brushing your teeth, or checking email. While you do this, scan your body for any sensations, tension, constriction, ease, softness. Just notice it and breathe into it. Then, go back to the activity, and then, back to your body. Over and over.

ONE BREATH AT A TIME

Breath, in many languages—*prana, chi, ruach*, also means "life force" or "spirit." It's that big and that important. As Etty Hillesum, who died in a Nazi concentration camp at twenty-nine years old, wrote in her diary, *Sometimes the most important thing in a whole day is the rest we take between two deep breaths.*

You instinctively take a big sigh, a long inhale, when you receive bad news or hear something hurtful, when there is too much to manage in a moment and your body instinctively creates space to hold it. You hold your breath when in fear or anticipation, or you take a deep breath if you are overwhelmed. The body is wise.

When you breathe deeply, you activate the ventral vagus nerve and signal your relaxation system to slow your heart rate and breath and turn on your digestion and restorative metabolic systems. The breath signals your body that it's time to *tend to* yourself. And that *you are safe*, in this moment. Your breath is a protector, your body's messaging system to *Turn down, take a pause.*

When meditators bring attention to their breath, they turn down that area of rumination, the default mode network, we have talked about, and get out of oppressive stories of the past and future to wander into connection, expansion, and openness. By learning to shine a light on your breath, you train yourself to focus on it as your way of being in a moment. Your body becomes your way of *seeing* the world.

Take a Pause

Think on it; when you breathe deeply, you don't only signal your relaxation system in your body. You also expand your body—widening your chest, moving your ribs, breathing into your belly—and occupy more space. Your breath can be your power move, harking back to Amy Cuddy's work.

Think of a time in the day you can offer to your breath, even if just for one to five minutes, a time you can remember to do it easily. Maybe right when you wake up (my favorite), before you go to sleep (especially if you have insomnia), before a workday starts, or one of my favorites, in a checkout line when otherwise my mind is prone to impatience and spinning into stories.

The power of your breath goes well beyond meditation or mindfulness. It can be your own guiding life force and touchstone on a path to Joy. Every time you return to your breath, you remind yourself of Justice-filled truth:

I am *capable of starting over in any one moment.*

I have the power to settle my activated nervous system.

I can release healing chemicals like oxytocin in my body that say I am safe, I am okay.

I open my chest where my heart resides, opening to the capacity to love and be loved.

I expand into space I was always entitled to occupy.

It is a tool that is often wholly underestimated. Free, accessible anytime, invisibly attended if need be. Noticing and tending to the breath may be the simplest and yet most powerful tool I teach. I tell my patients routinely when I, too, need a breath, if their stories have either overwhelmed my own nervous system or touched my heart so deeply that I need to open it wider to receive what I heard. I ask them to breathe with me so that they can feel the power the breath has to usher change.

If you are overwhelmed by your anger or sadness in any one moment, breathe into it and create space for more ease. Most acute emotions will pass through the body in a minute or two unless they get stuck, but the discomfort can be so great that we move to escape the sensation immediately. Try instead surfing the emotion like a wave; use your breath to *ride it out*. In this way, breath can be your friend, companion, and caregiver through uncomfortable moments.

The movement of your breath is a way to clear out the thick underbrush of your conditioned ways of being and thinking and instead, create flow and trust. Your body is always present. Now, how can you find *presence in your body*?

PRACTICE: BREATH AWARENESS

Paying attention to your breath is simple but not easy. It takes practice. This practice can be done anywhere, anytime, for a short time or longer. I love doing this upon awakening as a way to slow the urge to check my phone or start the doing of the day.

1. You can try something very simple to start. Close your eyes or settle your gaze softly ahead. Focus on your breath wherever is easiest, as you inhale through your nostrils or mouth, as it goes down the back of your throat, or as it is released. Breathe in for a count of two, hold and pause for two if able, and then exhale for four. You can change the amount but keep that rate of doubling your exhale to the equal counts of inhale and pause. The longer exhale gives our ventral vagal system a signal to relax even more. Try this and see how you feel in that moment but also after. I promise you, the power is exponential.
2. You can also try box breathing, which is widely known as the way US Navy SEALs improve concentration and calm in their work. This type of breath stimulates the vagus nerve and the parasympathetic system to decrease your heart rate and blood pressure. To start, exhale completely. Inhale slowly to a count of four, counting silently, letting the air fill your lungs and abdomen.

Hold your breath for a count of four. Then exhale for the same count of four. And once again hold the breath at the end of the exhale before starting again. Repeat for one to five minutes, or until you feel more calm in your body. Try to lengthen the time you spend noticing your breath by a bit each week.

UNTANGLING THE THREADS

I love you. I love this Brown skin that brought me into this world, has carried me, and protected me.

I was on a recliner in my own basement, but I might as well have been a thousand miles from home because this journey took me far from any usual resting place. I was serving as faculty in one of our mind body medicine trainings, but because of the 2020 COVID-19 pandemic, we had for the first time shifted to doing them virtually. The world at large was reeling from this viral pandemic and our country from its own overdue awakening to an ever-present epidemic of racism and injustice.

We were doing a body scan, an exercise in which you pay attention to each part, usually done from feet to head in sequence, and bring awareness to sensations in each area—tension, aches, or ease. This exercise had a twist. As we did the scan, to reverberating, rhythmic beats, we were prompted to not only travel our body but to ask it questions, to visit various organs and regions and see whether any unconscious wisdom or messages lay there. *Shoulder pain, what are you trying to tell me? Gut cramping, why are you so ever present?* Even though we were being led to various regions, I soon lost the voice of the guide as just background noise within the music. I found myself unable to leave a part of my body I had previously never visited: my skin.

I traveled underneath my skin, up and down, through my whole body. I could feel it from the outside and even from within, imagining the collagen layers and fascia underneath as if I was in some futuristic flight between each sheath. I stayed quiet and listened.

And then I heard a message, loud and clear.

I love you, I love you.... Over and over.

From my skin to my body and from my entire body to my skin.

I love you. I love this Brown skin that has brought me into this world, carried me, and protected me.

As I felt my skin from the inside out as beautiful, powerful, and wise, I recalled a painful truth—that I had spent too much time feeling shameful of my skin, wishing it was whiter, less hairy, smoother. But today, I felt an aliveness, a tingling feeling, and a freedom to roam my body without resistance. And so even when the music faded, I stayed reclined in that bliss for a few minutes more. I had not only listened with the full envelope of my skin, but I had also allowed that envelope to hold me.

As I lay there at the end, feeling so much Joy in my Brown body, that is when I clearly heard the phrase *Joy is my Justice.*

Pain lives in our body, but it can heal there too.

One day as I moved between warrior poses in a yoga class, I found myself getting bored and my mind wandering. Until I heard my teacher say, *feel into the pose*, and I found myself annoyed. *I'm standing in the pose, I want it to end; does that count?*

Breathe into your feet and feel them solidly taking up space on your mat.

Okay, I'll bite. *I feel my feet standing on this mat.*

I'm breathing.

I had stood in these poses countless times over. But today, I felt the arch of my foot wobbling along my soft mat, my thighs and hamstrings in counterstretch, my arms outstretched right to my fingers. And as she guided us to a plank pose and then a downward dog shape, I found myself instead retreating to child's pose, the prayerlike position in which you are folded over in ease, head down on mat, in surrender. And I could not move.

The rest of class moved on, but I lay there until I could see my brain inside my head, all the grooves and bumps. And then, I saw my brain wringing itself out like a dish towel, twisting on itself. Not painful but not altogether comfortable. And out of my brain, I saw anxiety, grief, frustration, anger, all dripping out with every twist onto my mat. I could see them flowing now, and they were endless. I got so lost in the image that I did not remember I was on my mat, until I felt how wet it was under my face. They had wrung themselves out in tears, pooling under me, having overflowed from a place that was too full to hold them any longer.

The evidence that trauma takes up residence in our autonomic nervous systems and can keep us in a hypervigilant state has been well proven by many, most notably by trauma expert Bessel van der Kolk, MD. He eloquently shows that the effects of past trauma literally live in your body and make it feel unsafe for you to inhabit it. The answer he gives is to cultivate a sense of safety in your body once again through a wide variety of therapies that eventually give you a sense of ease instead of hypervigilance. When you feel emotional pain in your body, you continue to scan your environment for harm until your body feels settled. You may have the experience or know others who have had to disassociate from their body to feel less pain and simply to survive. This isn't failure or weakness. It was their body caring for and protecting them; if you, too, had to dissociate, numb, or freeze in a situation, you did what you needed to do.

This happens not only on a whole body and nervous system level, as Dr. van der Kolk described. It occurs microscopically as well and is even termed, quite fittingly, in science as a *cell danger response*. Yes, that's right. Your cells find danger in your body—any inflammatory or infectious threat—and mount a healing response that can literally disconnect your cells in danger from the rest of your body to protect and heal them. This response can go on too long, even after the threat is no longer present, and be stored as *metabolic memory* in your cellular energy centers, the mitochondria. At all levels, your body is storing information, protecting you, and doing its best to mount a response or disconnect when needed.

Now can be the time to meet your body again and fine-tune your interoceptive awareness so that you can listen to what your body has learned and remembered over time. Yes, working with a professional is important, especially because often we are not aware of how much space trauma may occupy. But along with that, you can step lightly into your body over and over. Is it through dance, yoga, or running? Through walking or rolling, shaking or stretching as able? Think of it not as a scary place to meet your pain, but instead as a Justice-filled platform to find your power. The more you feel into your body and take up space within it, the more you can stand up in relation to others and to yourself.

PRACTICE: BODY SCAN

When you're ready to move on, it could be days or weeks, you can move to practicing attention in your body. You can also do this next exercise and the ones before in parallel to keep fine-tuning your awareness.

1. Get comfortable in a seated or lying down position.
2. Take a few deep breaths, close your eyes if able, and see whether you can find a bit more ease in your body.
3. Start at your feet and just notice, as if you are feeling them from the inside. Notice what bodily sensation(s) are most prominent for you.
4. Notice what this sensation feels like and whether it changes at all with your attention.
5. Spend one to three minutes attending to this sensation. If you notice thoughts or stories arise, gently either go back to the sensation or, if that is too challenging, take a break and notice your breath.
6. Travel slowly from your feet upward to your calves, thighs, pelvis, and on. Go to whichever parts of your body you like. There is no order that is right. The practice is done traditionally from toe to head or in reverse merely for simplicity and to take the planning part out of the practice. You can do this exercise as such or add the next steps as well. Your choice.

7. After a few minutes on any part of your body, you can widen your focus to your body as a whole, maybe even giving it gratitude for whatever messages it gives you. Spend a few moments noticing your body as a whole.
8. Come back to the sensation and notice how it feels now. It might be the same or have changed a bit.
9. Keep cycling from a sensation to your body as a whole. Go through as many parts of your body as able or desired.
10. After five to fifteen minutes or when you feel done, breathe a few deep breaths and open your eyes.
11. If this exercise feels too challenging, no problem. You can instead slow down with any daily activity and just practice paying attention. Maybe to washing dishes or cooking. Notice your hands and how it feels to touch the objects, what the ground beneath you feels like, the sounds; just notice. This mindful slowing down can help fine-tune your interoceptive awareness.

HOPE MOLECULES

I was in another fishbowl group exercise, a smaller circle like the one I had once sat in, again surrounded by larger concentric rings. But this time, I was the one leading it. I was in Northern California's Shasta County, coleading a program for the communities traumatized by the devastating wildfires of 2018. We happened to hold the training in graciously offered church space, but the circle would have been sacred all the same when six individuals offered to be in the middle of the room and work even deeper to meet their pain.

Justin, a leader in this relatively small community and now a volunteer in the fishbowl, shared how challenging it was to hold this community's pain while tending to his. Devastation, emotional and physical, surrounded him. Amid it all, he teetered a delicate balance of being a beacon of hope and, on this day, human enough to admit his had waned. This often led to him feeling that he was *not enough*, he admitted. The tenderness in his sharing was powerful and I found myself seeing reflections of familiar disappointment.

The exercise I chose to do in this small group was a shaking meditation of the body, followed by a couple of minutes of silence, and then some free movement, or dancing. Shaking meditation is a tool as old as time itself, respectfully borrowed from traditions across the globe, as ancient as the whirling dervishes and Indigenous shamanic healers, and in my estimation, demands the respect of its endurance. It is a movement meditation that allows you to literally *shake it out* and get to emotions that are bubbling just underneath the surface and hungry to move. Movement is one of the core ways to complete a stress cycle. Animals do it intuitively in the wild after escaping a predator and shake out their fear. Humans often neglect completing the cycle due to hurried life or avoidance.

All in the circle shared, we did the shaking meditation, and then came back to check in on what came up in that experience. When it was Justin's turn, he looked at me, put a hand on his heart, and smiled. He described his *strange experience*, that usually he dreads dancing. *It's my wife who can't get off the dance floor.* Being self-conscious already and then in this large room felt like a challenge. But he found himself slowly but surely releasing anxiety and tension through his shaking body for several minutes, until he started to feel tingling in his hands and an energy of Joy. Then, a thought emerged as well: *I am banging it out here!* He started to laugh, wondering whether how good a dancer he was in that moment was only in the magic of his own mind or a reality. He even opened his eyes for a second to assure himself this was a real moment.

A seemingly small, Joyful moment, but so much more in there. Hope, release, freedom.

The larger group had a good chuckle with him and then as there was silence yet again, I asked of him, *And how did it feel to be good enough?*

He smiled, tapped his heart gently with his palm. *So fun, so good.*

In that one small moment, Justin offered a reflection of what we all so desperately want. To feel free in our body, to feel Joy in even a small moment, and to feel like that is enough. No lofty expectations of us, no answers we need to have. Just the feeling of comfort in our own body. Right here, right now.

As you meet your body and learn to move it, so, too, can you meet the pain and then learn to move that. Movement of any kind can be the antidote to the freeze and stuckness you may be feeling; it can help you move *forward and with* your life. It is also a powerful drug in the brain, stimulating what is called our endocannabinoid receptor system that makes us feel pleasure and even the high some people identify. Moving your body also makes this system more sensitive so that when you stimulate the receptors used to bond with others, it can feel better each time. *You feel even more Joy.* Movement also increases a sophisticated neurochemical in the brain called brain-derived neurotrophic factor (BDNF), which helps us improve memory and learning, among other things. And it's not just about your biochemistry. Movement is primal and awakens you to your body, the vessel that carries you forward each day, even when your mind doubts you can.

Take a Pause

Think about that. Movement increases both feel-good hormones and BDNF. Your body can feel Joy and then, *remember* and *learn from* this moment so the next boost of Joy is even stronger.

I have a fondness for shaking, this ancient tool of expressive meditation, because it not only releases stuck emotions but also gives us a chance to reset our nervous system. I never know what I will experience, at times utter freedom and lightness in my body and at others, tension, tears of grief, or heaviness—emotions and sensations that literally *move* into their next version. I couldn't agree more with holistic psychiatrist Ellen Vora, MD, author of *The Anatomy of Anxiety*, who describes this reset: *Shaking is like pressing <ctrl-alt-delete>... this appears to tell the nervous system, in an old and hard-wired manner, that the threat has passed, and you are now safe.* You complete that stress cycle and turn off hyper-vigilant watch. When I get to the silence part, before I release myself into dance, I almost always feel a reassuring tingling in my hands, the reminder that energy has moved and that I am alive enough to feel it. Whether I find myself in tears, or at other times, laughter, it's all living right under my envelope, waiting to be met. E-motions are energy in motion, so this kind of movement allows them to work through me.

Notice I don't use the word *exercise*, but *movement*. This is not about measuring your steps or losing weight. I am talking about survival. Put simply, moving your body is part of your toolkit to withstand the brutality of this world. It could be running, spinning, or shaking in your wheelchair. I have shaken with patients who are lying in their hospital bed. We can all move gently toward the freedom our body needs in any one moment.

I don't doubt that the music component of this shaking meditation is part of the magic. Music does literally move you, lighting up the motor cortex, priming your muscles to spring into action. It stimulates dopamine and endorphins and literally moves your emotions through chemistry. Music also moves you quickly to memories in your body, both Joyous and heartbreaking. Turn on a Counting Crows song and I am right back in one of my most painful breakups. And if you turn on any Janet Jackson track from *Rhythm Nation 1814*, I can transport faster than you can blink to an outdoor concert in Chicago with one of my best friends from college. I instantly feel young, free, and so firmly in my body, dancing like that warm summer evening outside in balmy Midwest air.

This is all why I suggest turning on music of their choice to my depressed patients who can hardly get out of bed. I urge them to listen every day until it moves them to take one small movement forward. And then hope for another. Muscles actually produce myokines, anti-inflammatory messengers that scientists themselves call *Hope molecules*. And any movement, no matter how small, produces this hope. That inspires me. Your thoughts get in the way and say you cannot do something, but then your body not only proves you wrong but whispers, *Trust yourself, you are bigger than this.*

PRACTICE: SHAKING AND DANCING MEDITATION

Yes, this exercise can feel a bit weird the first time you try it, but trust me, it is worth getting past the skepticism. I routinely do it in groups, and in those cases, have people close eyes, turn toward a wall to turn down self-consciousness, or hold on to something for balance. Also, if it feels too strange for you, by all means, let any music of your choice move you as your meditation. There is no dictum of how to move. I have seen powerful results using the meditation in this way. And if you choose to do all three parts of the meditation, I list them out here. But as I said, choose just the shaking, the free movement at the end, or your own movement of choice. This is your Joy journey.

1. Part 1: roughly five to seven minutes of shaking. Plant your feet on the floor if you are able, but if you need to, do this in a seat or lying down. All and any shaking is good. Close eyes to go more inward if you choose. Do what you need though for balance.
2. Plant your feet firmly on ground if you are standing, give a soft bend in your knees, and shake up through your body as you choose.
3. Choose whatever rhythmic, deep beats you feel safe with. I often use drumming music for its repetitive and resounding

rhythm. Most important, for this portion, use music without lyrics so you are not swept up into those and can stay in your body.

4. Part 2: After this, stand (or sit or lay) still for one to two minutes. Just notice what you feel in your body and heart.
5. Part 3: And then turn on music of your choice and let the music move you as you wish.
6. At the end, notice how and what you feel as compared to when you started. Try using this daily or a few times a week and see what emerges for you. I like using it after a long workday or to move energy in the morning.

YOUR RHYTHMS

I'm the furthest thing from a Deadhead, or so I thought.

Steve will tell you defiantly that his love for the Grateful Dead has very little to do with the drugs and everything to do with the community and how it reminds him of core truths of humanity. He can tear up instantly if you even bring up the song "Broke-down Palace." Play a live version of it and the tears come in less than a nanosecond.

Mama, mama, many worlds I've come since I first left home....

Through all life's changes, the Grateful Dead have been his constant and this line reminds him each time that their music brings him home to his body, to the essence of what he loves and what is best in him. *You can leave your wallet on the ground at a concert, and it will be there hours later when you come back,* he loves to tell me. Deadheads care for one another and when he is with them, he always feels cared for. I think it has everything to do with sharing music in community, moving and singing together to one harmonic vibration. The neuroscience tells us that this kind of movement puts us *in sync* with others and floods us with neurochemicals of Joy and connection like serotonin, dopamine, and oxytocin. The music makes us want to be closer to one another.

When they sang the last lines of the song, it was almost always as an encore that he describes as a love letter from the band to the crowd and the crowd back to the band in reciprocal gratitude for this shared time.

Fare you well, fare you well.

I love you more than words can tell....

After he dries his tears, Steve reminisces with me about that moment: *You could always feel the same exact emotion vibrating through the crowd... love.*

The Dead are not my jam, but even I tear up when he tells me this. I feel that same belonging and connection when I share my traditional dance of Bhangra in community, like the most rapid booster of bliss I can find. Our music and dance are like nothing else (I know I'm biased, but attend a Punjabi wedding and you'll never be the same): intergenerational unison of footwork and clapping, rhythmic drums, singing and outright howling with one another, and circles of dancing and laughter. And if I dance to the music, at home or even in my car, it can take me right back to my favorite celebratory memories and then to Joy faster than nothing else. I think Steve and I are both experiencing the same thing. When you move, and with others, you not only feel good, you want to reach out and be closer to them. You want to care for others and yourself. *You feel more. Alive.*

My theory as well is that as humans, we want so badly to expand from our constricted patterns and sense of self. We fiercely want to be bigger and freer than the small stories life has painted for us. Movement, music, and even psychedelic medicine all do this by dampening that default mode network and taking us out of our habitual rumination and worry to an expanded perception of self and others. And if this shared movement is outside in nature, then it can be even more amplified. Even just one ninety-minute walk in nature had this effect, as seen on a functional MRI. And a walk among trees can literally decrease your stress hormones and downregulate your nervous system as you inhale their soothing chemicals. The trees literally care for you. It's no wonder why a summer group walk to raise money for brain cancer can make me feel rejuvenated instead of depressed. Movement in community makes you feel that you belong to something greater because you have expanded yourself beyond the narrow confines of the space you inhabited before.

This year, my family and I joined forty-five-plus others along the Camino de Santiago in Spain, a heavily tread pilgrimage in the name of Saint James, with the group I'll Push You, who organize accessible group Caminos. We had six captains, as they were called, individuals in wheelchairs, including Zubin. They rolled as able; we pushed, pulled, and walked alongside them.

One of my clearest images from that Camino was the Spanish policemen who tried to stop us from going down an incredibly steep Roman road when they saw our wheels and feet approaching. *No puedes ir allí. No es para sillas de ruedas.* (You can't go there.

It's not for wheelchairs.) But go we did. And to anyone's knowledge, there have never been wheelchairs that have rolled down that road and Zubin would be by far the youngest to ever do so. So, yes, there was a sense of physical accomplishment among the whole group and that is emotional on its own. But there was more than just this outdoor movement to create such a flow of emotions.

Those six days, we shared the purpose of a common goal. We shared awe for one another, for these captains and what they were accomplishing now but also what they had endured daily in their lives. And each day, we moved our body as we moved into one another's story. We had built community and connection around belief and those Hope molecules, not just that we could accomplish anything we put our body's attention to, but that *together* we were moving with more strength and purpose than any one of us could alone. When we all entered that final point, the square in Santiago de Compostela, there was not a dry eye in the group.

If movement can release emotions and untangle what is stuck, consider this. Moving in rhythm, and with others, may unleash the larger potential of the collective power we hold. Maybe you, too, like Steve, have felt this power at a dance party or concert, where everyone was synchronously vibrating to the same song, maybe even singing it in unison. I instantly think of being in my hometown of New Orleans during Mardi Gras and dancing to parade drum lines with throngs of people. It reverberates through your body in a way you cannot achieve alone.

Find *your* Justice, your rhythm. The science stands that when you move through rhythm, it *moves you* to feel better, perseverate less on the more difficult nuances of the stories of your life, and be more *a part of* this world than *apart from* it.

YOUR BODY MAKES SENSE

A few years after Zubin's diagnosis, I took a pottery class at a local clay studio, something I had never even thought of trying before. But I knew deep in my bones that I needed to get my hands on something. I couldn't make any sense of my world and so I had to make sense of something from the earth itself.

I went to that studio every week and created things. I stayed quiet the entire class, every week. Never said a thing. No one knew I was a doctor, that my son was dying, that I was desperate to put my hands around something real. I just went and made things.

And I started healing. Because healing is not fixing; it is knowing what you feel so that you can feel into that. Knowing that when you can still make something, anything, you undeniably exist. *Making* is the body's antidote when the mind does not know what to *do.*

Take a Pause

What creative outlet gives you Joy? Is there one that puts you in a *flow* state? Or is there one that has called to you? I found two new and surprising ones in the pandemic—calligraphy and urban sketching. Both helped me manage my anxiety. You never know where your next creative ground will be—the earth, flowers, a pen, paintbrush, clay, food.

I met a woman once who had lost both her children in a horrific accident. She was so taken by her grief that she left her work in health care and made mosaics with pieces of glass. Because making something beautiful and whole out of shards of broken earth spoke to her. She then opened her studio to others who needed to work through pain by moving their hands and creating. Sometimes in silence, sometimes in community. If you ask me, she did not leave the profession of healing, she merely expanded it.

Sylvia came into the clinic, ostensibly to address her worsening back pain. But when I asked her about stress in her life, she began to cry and admitted that she was days away from the anniversary of her son's death. And now that she thought about it, at this time of the year, she often feels more depressed and has more pain. I asked her what she had planned to do on his birthday and she almost chuckled. *Probably the same thing as every year: stay in my apartment alone and cry.*

I asked her a simple question: *What do you think your body needs on that day?* Together, we explored that concept—she needed, she said, to feel less alone—and designed a ritual that felt right to her. This year, she would go to the lake—her son loved to swim and be by the water any chance he could. She would bake him a small cake because that was their birthday ritual. She would cut the cake in his honor by the water, and cry there instead, surrounded by what he loved and eating what they loved together.

When you perform or attend a ritual, the rest of life is silent while you take it in. I remember exactly the look on my mother's face at my wedding after Steve and I took our last turn around our holy book, signifying the marriage was sealed. She was right there with me, transfixed. Ritual brings you into your body, anchoring you to what is going on right here, in the now, whether the moments are joyous or sad.

The neuroscience supports that even small rituals offer a piece of certainty each time. In sports, they are often used to decrease anxiety and have some small amount of predictability before a game. Huddling around one another and doing the same chants, entering the court a specific way, all these things create a small amount of assurance where there is none. You can assign more meaning to a ritual by simply calling it one rather than experiencing it as a random act. Sylvia later told me that saying to herself this is how she was honoring both her son *and* her grief made it a more meaningful day to her than staying at home and letting the day be, as she described it, *empty*. She gave herself a small piece of Justice when the tragedy could offer none.

Take a Pause

You hear so much in the self-empowerment world about the importance of having a morning ritual. It feels, to me, like a teaching that is offered in a very *military-tough-win-the-day* type of tone. The science is clear that a morning (or any time of day) ritual can be helpful. But let's soften the approach. This routine is not to *win* anything but to *come back to yourself, to give your body a soft place to land when the world feels too hard, to assure yourself even though life may not be okay, you are okay, right here, right now, in this moment.*

We can't only make sense of the world through our minds. It is through our body that we create meaning when there seems to be none. We make things—art, food, rituals—no matter how large or small. We come to the moment through our whole envelope and hold what we have until we make enough sense to hold more.

CHAPTER 10

Hope for Yourself

IS THERE HOPE?

Hope is your quiet revolution that knows this story can change. It's your lifeline, your birthright. Hope is:

Bold action in the face of despair.

Your fight for a better day than the one in front of you.

Yours to have and no one's to take away.

Self-love in action; your body's deepest knowing that you are worthy.

The conviction that not only are you here, but you *deserve* to be here.

The deepest antidote to the unworthiness that oppression bestows on us.

The question is not, *Is there hope?* The question is, *How can you harness the hope already inside you to once again meet the world that tried to erase it?*

HOPE SEES THE UNSEEN

I was shuttling from patient to patient on a busy clinic afternoon, obsessively glancing at my pager. My day got more frayed by the minute as I waited for a call while, at the same time, I hoped it never came.

It was my second year of residency, and I now had a panel of my own patients in clinic, whose care felt like a weighty responsibility in my young hands. The day before, I had visited with a new patient, Mrs. Kao. Something about her reassuring smile made me feel as if we had known each other for much longer. When she first explained her shortness of breath, she downplayed the severity. She had put off coming to the doctor ever since her prior family physician had retired.

But Mrs. Kao had been short of breath for a few months now, and it was affecting her ability to walk the steep hills of her Seattle neighborhood and disrupting her favorite pastime, gardening. In between her medical history, she let me into more of her life story. She was widowed and alone, her two children living out of town. She was fiercely independent, so much so that even coming to the doctor for help was out of her ordinary.

I did a thorough physical exam and some labs. Her breath sounds were normal but there was a sound in her heart I had never heard before, which signaled that I might need help. My favorite cardiologist in the hospital somehow had a slot open for the next day and I was able to get her in. When he took time out of his busy schedule to page me at lunchtime, I knew it was a bad sign.

Tanmeet, Mrs. Kao has a large pericardial effusion. I am admitting her to the hospital until I can get free this evening to drain it. If I didn't have even more urgent procedures lined up, I would do it now.

In lay terms, this means that she had fluid hugging her heart in all the wrong and tightest ways. And even though he was booked all afternoon with other emergency procedures, she was too risky to send home without monitoring or to wait even one more day. So now, after a casual start to our relationship, things got dicey, very quickly. The possibility of a scary outcome—if the fluid got too large or tight around the heart, she could have a cardiac arrest—as she waited for the procedure preoccupied me as I sat with other patients.

After I was done with clinic, I raced up to the hospital to see her. When I walked in her room, she was sitting up on a bed with the back fully propped up. She was breathing quicker than yesterday, her chest rising and falling noticeably even through her hospital gown, but her face still with the same calm as when I first met her in my exam room. She looked at me, then the clock on the wall, and smiled.

It's late. You must be tired.

I flushed at the thought of her worrying about *me.*

I'm fine. I'm worried about you, I said as I sat by the side of her bed.

We talked about her children, her garden, but most important, about her hope.

Hope in this situation seemed foreign to me. I had just come out of medical school training where the dictum from my attending physicians was not to ever give our patients *false hope.* That in some way, we would then be downplaying the seriousness of their condition and then they would too. It was as if hope could be risky.

So, here I was, a young physician with so much fear. For my patient. For the worst possible outcome.

I asked whether she was scared. She didn't hesitate.

Yes, but there's always hope. Always.

She took my hand in hers, squeezed it in reassurance, and went on. *And Dr. Sethi, the upside of hope is too big to let it slip away.* She had seen too much suffering in her life to not believe hope was the right and best thing to do. That evening, in a dimly lit, sterile hospital room, I had the seeds sown that hope could live without relying on anyone or anything but your own persistent desire to have it.

Barack Obama wrote a book called *The Audacity of Hope*. Confession: I still haven't read it, but the title alone stirs me. Yes, President Obama, it is audacious to have hope. It is a bold act of Justice. No one should ever be able to decide *for* you when hope is permissible. Mind you, I'm writing this in the midst of a seemingly never-ending pandemic, a rapidly rising climate crisis, and on the heels of a presidential administration that stirred a vigilance in me like never before. All made even more stressful by a growing divisiveness in this country, an intensity of which I have never seen in my lifetime. There are days when I feel beaten down, scared, and even spiral into existential crisis over where we are headed. And I wonder then whether I can have that audacity.

For Zubin, there is certainly no hope in the conventional sense, certainly none that my medical school teachers would see. He has a fatal disease, and before the end, things are getting much worse. The first physician to sit us down to give us his genetic fate apologized: *There is nothing we can do; I am so sorry.* His shattering words still reverberate through my heart. I wish then he knew what I know now.

Hope is exactly how you are still able to get up every day, no matter what has come on the one before. It lives in your actions even when you don't recognize it and gives birth to both the small steps and large movements. Bryan Stevenson, one of my activist idols and founder of Equal Justice Initiative, advocates against the industrial prison complex, our modern-day version of slavery. When my mind overtakes my body's natural impulse to hope, I remember his words. *I think my hope is not entirely rational... it's just rooted in this belief that truth crushed to earth ultimately rises again. I don't think you can do this work if you're unwilling to believe things you haven't seen*, he says.

His words awakened my insight that I was too *scared* to voice hope amid tragedy. That I, too, thought I needed some logic or proof to support it. But the most powerful move I can make today is to hold hope whether others believe I should or not. I hope, every day now, for even more than a cure. I hope for moments of ease, dignity, and strength; for love to surround my son and family every day; for his brother and sister to learn that the value of our lives is not based on the length or what we can achieve, but how we live and love. I want to go back to Zubin's first doctor and say, *No, there is so much we can do. So much to hope for.* Even doctors with grim news and predictions cannot take that away.

Hope is always *something* I can do. Even if a fair outcome seems unlikely, the right to hope is my own Justice, in my body, where it matters most. I speak not only as a Justice activist. We *all* need something to keep fighting for, in our lives. Hope is a powerful arsenal *to stay alive* in this often exhausting and depressing world.

Hope protects your brain, in the most loving way, even if the hope is merely for fear to not overtake you. And when you move away from hope, you go closer to despair. I didn't realize it then, but Mrs. Kao gave me my first lesson in the neuroscience of hope, untangling the disempowering teaching I had received in medical school.

My patient, Carla, a healthy and active woman in her forties, came in complaining of some persistent leg pain. After further evaluation, we found what neither of us could have ever expected: a growing sarcoma, a tumor engulfing her thigh muscle. When she came in to get the results, she slumped down the wall onto the floor. We sat in silence together as she cried, and even when we talked about next steps, fear, understandably, still took up much of the space in that room.

Before Carla left, I put my hand on my heart. *I will hold hope for you until you can hold it for yourself.* Until she could feel its strong vibration coursing through her body.

There is always room for hope.

For the yet unseen.

PRACTICE: THE MUSCLE OF HOPE

To ground in hope, you can first practice grounding in your own body. This reminds you how stable your body can be, and then, by extension, as you practice, you gain more stability in your mind and heart. This practice reminds you how easily you can hold hope for others, that your hope muscle already exists.

I like doing this exercise either seated or standing with my feet planted on the ground. If this does not work for you, you can sit or lie in any position that feels comfortable to you. No matter what position you assume, I want you to feel the support of the earth, seat, or bed beneath you. And if you are able, lower your gaze or even close your eyes.

1. Start by taking a few deep breaths. Notice your breath where it feels most prominent. As it comes in your mouth or nostrils, as it goes down the back of your throat, maybe as it expands your lungs or belly, or on its way out. Wherever that is for you, be with your breath as you inhale and exhale. Inhale and exhale.
2. Now, try to lengthen the exhale a bit. Try inhaling for a count of two and exhaling for a count of four or six. Continue this way for a few more breaths, inhaling and exhaling for longer. As you breathe in and out, feel the support and stability underneath you. You are held in this moment. If you are standing or sitting with your feet on the ground, imagine roots from your feet extending out into the earth. If you are in a seat or bed, imagine these coming from the base of your spine.
3. Now, with your body supported, direct your breath to the space around your heart, continuing to breathe in and out. Imagine in your heart's eye someone in this life whom you love dearly. As you breathe into your heart, feel it expand, and then

breathe out the energy of your heart toward them. Notice how this feels in your body.

4. Imagine a time when this person you love so dearly has hoped for something or struggled in their life. A time when you wished only the very best for them. It doesn't have to be their biggest struggle; something easier will be a good way to start. See whether you can re-create your hope for them in your heart right now. How much you wished for their highest good, their best outcome. Notice how easily this hope may flow into your heart.
5. As you breathe in, breathe in their hope. As you breathe out and feel your heart expand, send your hope to them. Let this cycle of hope continue as you inhale and exhale and let it amplify. Let hope expand your heart even more. Give yourself a few minutes to feel this expansion.

FALSE HOPE IS THE LIE

Hope is never false.

When I heard one of my Integrative Medicine mentors say that, I felt its simple but bold truth land deep in my bones. I had confused this delusion of false hope with false positivity or even optimism, but they are all different. Hope cannot be a false construct. By definition, it must first acknowledge today's reality. When we hope, we are not *thinking positive*, we are instead acknowledging the deep despair we feel right now.

People tend to use *hope* and *optimism* as synonyms, but that isn't accurate. Optimism is believing things will be okay and studies show there is health benefit in that, yes, as compared to pessimism. Hope as well has been shown to improve well-being, heart health, and even success at work. One study parsed out the two concepts. It determined that *hope focuses more directly on the personal attainment of specific goals, whereas optimism focuses more broadly on the expected quality of future outcomes in general.* In other words, hope makes no assumption that things will be okay; it is instead personal action to make even one small aspect better today.

Hope may be the truest, most innate gift we have. It is powerful and steadfast and not dependent on a belief that life always works out because for many of us, it simply has not. Hope is the conviction that there is a reason to keep fighting because we choose to see what others cannot.

REMOVE THE CONDITIONS

I asked one of the resident physicians I train how their fellowship interview went.

Good, I think, but I don't want to get my hopes up.

Why not, why wouldn't you have hope?

Their predictable answer: to prevent disappointment if the outcome was a rejection.

Won't you be disappointed, no matter what, if you are rejected?

Well, of course.

Then, why spend more time in disappointment?

Take a Pause

Notice for yourself next time where fear resides in your body. Your shoulders, your jaw, your heart...? When you don't *want to get your hopes up*, where do you brace or constrict? Can you allow hope to share the moment and open you up to more of the possible, more than just the smaller story your fear has written for you?

What if, just what if, you found *unconditional hope*?

Hope is simply good for your health. It has been linked to happiness, less physical pain, and is even a strong predictor of mortality, especially if you have a threatening illness. In fact, in one study of three hundred–plus middle-aged patients scheduled to undergo coronary artery bypass surgery, those who believed in their good outcome were only half as likely to require rehospitalization!

Hope, to me, is the foundation of the placebo effect in research. You take a pill or try a treatment that hypothetically could help, and your entire body wants that to be true. So, even though you are not receiving the actual treatment, your body acts as if it has. It believes and wants to see what is possible. This effect, present as much as half the time, remains a mystery. It seems to be a complex mix of neurotransmitters and changes in the brain that give the body the stimulus to heal. I'll call it biologic Justice myself.

I'll as well give you the part that hasn't been studied but has come, instead from my decades of taking care of patients and being a mama. *When you have hope, you are open and expansive, in your body's power pose.*

I noticed, over a decade ago, as I was fighting for school inclusion for Zubin, that I would go into each meeting wishing to be hopeful but instead, deep down inside, not *wanting to get my hopes up*. And I would brace, I would constrict (mostly in my neck and shoulders), and I could feel this tension mount inside me as I neared the meeting day.

When you move away from hope, you invariably move toward negative thinking. Moreover, you lose the opportunity to carve new paths in your brain. Each time I or that resident physician resists hope, we expect less.

Your brain is biased to look for the negative, the threats. Why not live more of those moments leading up to the decision in the possible, in feeling the full expanse of hope? When you wait in hope, you carve new grooves in your brain—and even if the answer is a disappointment, you have primed your brain for living more time in the *possible*. In the *unseen*.

Take a Pause

The next time you're wanting to be hopeful for something or someone but feel scared to do so, take a moment, stop, and remember this: If you can't hope, what is there left? And if you don't get what you were hoping for, what have you lost? Find your own authentic way to hold hope close: *I am scared, but today I choose hope. Hope is never false. Hope is always with me.*

Hope is a great balancer in life. Things are so hard and then you harness hope that there can be better, that there is that featherbed on the other side. You let that balance all the fear, anger, and grief of the moment.

My oldest son was considering auditioning for the city's youth symphony, the most competitive one for his age. One day, he revealed he had changed his mind, and when I asked why, it was because a music teacher had told him he *wouldn't make it*. I was pissed. Not because I cared about the orchestra, but because this teacher had just shattered his hope. Even if it was what they believed, they could have followed it up with a truthful statement, that no one can predict the outcome or that the act of even trying may be a worthwhile practice in itself. I explained why now he *had* to audition. Just to *practice* hope. No one, no teacher, physician, or parent, has the right to take that away.

THE KINDLING

In February 2022, Russia launched a full-scale attack against Ukraine. It wasn't its first time to incite unrest there, but it was the most brutal show of force yet. The world spoke back. Protests, donations, refugee assistance. Anything to support Ukraine's efforts to sustain their land and lives. So, I did not hesitate at the opportunity in June of the same year to work with 150 Ukrainian citizens, mostly psychiatrists and psychologists, on the ground, living through the war while still attending to their people's traumas as they unfolded. It was a two-day virtual emergency response to teach them mind body medicine skills for their community and also for themselves.

Despite my existential distress when that training ended, that I had the privilege of turning off my computer and going back to my safe home while they had to yet endure, they gifted me a powerful and persistent lesson about hope. This war in Ukraine had felt like yet another blow in the long onslaught of tragedies the world was doling out. An ongoing pandemic, oppressive regimes globally, climate disasters throughout, social unrest. The fight was never ending and now there was one more to wage. And at times, I admit attending protests left me with less hope instead of more. *What was the point? Was anyone listening?*

But to a person, even with air strikes overhead, disrupting their Wi-Fi and psyches, the participants were steadfast in their gratitude to the world at large, for the *support* they felt and the encouragement with the protests. *We feel like we are not alone. It gives us hope.*

It occurred to me that the world's protesting and demanding of change couldn't only be measured in the desired outcome, although that was still the unified goal. Our show of hope was also fundamental to *their* well of hope. Our belief that they deserved better kindled their faith as well. None of us *saves* anyone. But our hope can help sustain one another's revolution.

I spent time with the community of Marjory Stoneman Douglas High School in 2018, five short months after a young shooter killed seventeen people and wounded seventeen more. My colleagues and I were invited to attend to the unspeakable trauma that students, teachers, parents, and community members had endured. On the third day of the workshop, in my small group of ten, something clicked for one teacher. *I'm at the same time so relieved and incredibly pissed off. Why hadn't anyone taught us these kinds of exercises right away? No one knew what to do for us*, she practically yelled. Others in the group nodded in return.

No, she was not suddenly all healed in that moment. But she still says to me, years later, that those five days *opened me up*. In her words, she *now had hope*. And that energy of hope awakened the belief that her healing could continue. *She was able to see the unseen*. In so many possible forms, from sweet gratitude to fiery anger, hope is the kindling to your revolution.

CHAPTER 11

Gratitude Doesn't Solve Everything

NOT GRATITUDE, AGAIN

Gratitude is one of those words that deserves a bit of a disclaimer before we go on. There are T-shirts, coffee shop slogans, celebs, and self-help experts who tell us to be grateful, to find the silver lining, and to stay positive. It's just one more task on the long list of things we're supposed to practice *to make things better.*

But gratitude is not a wishy-washy platitude. It doesn't solve everything or mask reality. It is about looking at life, instead of away, and finding the sliver of this moment that feels like something worth living and fighting for. Gratitude fundamentally shifts biochemistry and puts you in an awareness state to make change. It's on par in changing neurochemistry and immunology with tools like exercise or high-intensity interval training. It's real science and magic all the same. And it may be one of the most powerful tools for healing through oppression and suffering that I know.

FACE THE RIGHT DIRECTION

Gratitude solidly lands you in your body where the healing needs to happen. When you say *thank you* for something, you arrive into your life instead of escaping it. *Thank you for this job, this friend, this cup of coffee.* And it doesn't count to be grateful for the woes you don't have, but to be specifically grateful for what you *do*. Studies show that people who do something as simple as keep a gratitude journal, noting one to three things a day they're grateful for, feel better, sleep deeper, get sick less often, and even have more hope for life. Just by noting something they appreciate every day. This might be one of the simplest yet most consistent prescriptions I give to patients.

Take a Pause

Right now, pause and think of one thing to be grateful for. This is the simple seed of a powerful gratitude practice.

Julie was struggling with a depressed mood, unemployment, and hopelessness. So, we added this practice to her other treatments. Her gratitude journal went something like this:

Day 1: *Getting up, warm coffee, going back to bed*

Day 2: *Getting up, warm coffee, sitting in the sunlight from the window*

Day 3: *Warm coffee, walking around the block, a smile from a neighbor*

Day 4: *Warm coffee, having a brief moment of laughter with a friend, flowers on a walk*

And so on for a month. It may not sound that revolutionary. She, too, wondered at first whether it was silly or whether she had enough to write about. *Is it really okay to count coffee that many days in a row?* she asked me. But then she found it wasn't actually *what* she wrote that felt like a shift.

The biggest thing I noticed was that I was asking a question all day: Could this be something I am grateful for tonight? It wasn't that I was looking for things but instead I was looking at things in a different way.

That, to me, is a revolution. The same life looks different. This may seem easy when you're thankful for good things (although I would argue nothing looks good when you're depressed), but the bigger question is how or even why to be grateful when things are challenging. Let's break gratitude down a bit more first.

There are a couple of tweaks that seem to uplevel this practice, such as sharing this gratitude daily with someone (I suggest out loud, but if not, even by email or text) and being specific about why you're grateful (add *because* to the end of your gratitude—really spell it out) for something or someone. For example, instead of *I am grateful for Steve . . . I am grateful for Steve because he makes me laugh every day no matter what.*

The science suggests that the more you express gratitude, the more it acts as an anti-inflammatory molecule to make your immune system stronger, the more neurochemicals—serotonin and dopamine—you secrete to make you happier, and it acts as a messenger in your nervous system to decrease the resting state of your fear centers. Every time Julie asked her question, she calmed the center of her brain that looked for threat instead.

Gratitude changes your physiology. It directly decreases your heart rate in the same way as when your body relaxes and feels safe. The science even shows that people with heart failure do better just by noting a few things they are grateful for daily. *Let me say that again: gratitude makes your heart work better.*

The science also shows that the stronger your practice gets, not only can you feel more ease with your past painful experiences, but you can inoculate yourself against future trauma. When things are hard in your life, gratitude can feel so very challenging. But remember that you are not denying the bad or hard, you are widening your lens, so you *don't forget the good.* As you see these nourishing parts of your world, you reclaim your power instead of giving more away.

PRACTICE: PATHS TO DAILY GRATITUDE

1. Many cultures and traditions have a ritual of saying thanks before eating. For good reason: It puts you in more of a parasympathetic state, helping you digest and absorb your food. It can also be a source of connection to the world. Here is a variation on this type of gratitude practice: Express thanks for your meal while tracing how you received this food. You might want to thank the sun, rain, and wind that grew this food, marveling at the wonders of this Earth. Thank the farmers who toiled the land and harvested the crops or the factory workers who packaged the food, the drivers who transported it to the store, the cashiers who sold it to you, whoever cooked it for you, and on and on. In one bite, you could see the web of your

intricate connection to the Earth and even others you will never meet but who made this moment possible.

2. Another one of my favorite ways to practice gratitude is with a *gratitude jar*. This is a jar (or any container) you can put anywhere in your home or work and have small pieces of paper next to it. Whenever someone feels moved, they can write down a gratitude, fold the paper, and place it in the jar. You can have a set time you or your family pull notes out of the jar to read together. We used to do this at Sunday dinners a couple of times a month. It was a reminder of the good that we may have passed by or forgotten. Or you can pull them out on the spot for a Joy booster. I have had countless patients do this in their homes or resident physicians have put jars in the hospital team room.

SWIM IN IT

It was 2011, in a shuttle van to the airport and the rain was unrelenting. My husband and I said not a word the whole ride. Zubin sat in between us, looking as stunned. It felt like we had just been through a hailstorm. Tests, X-rays, several doctors, nine hours in the Cincinnati Children's Hospital. And none of the news was good.

There was no treatment program for DMD at our local children's hospital at the time and our insurance had generously agreed to pay for visits to one of the only clinical centers in the country. And we took the plunge, grateful for the privilege to afford the trip, but made it quick for our kids at home. One night in, a full day of doctors and tests, and now, home, as fast as possible. Where there was no treatment program for our son. Not knowing at all what this life would look like.

When we reached the airport, the shuttle driver who had also sat in complete silence with us headed to the trunk to get our luggage. My husband got out a tip and handed it to him.

Oh no, please, for trips from the children's hospital, I don't take tips. It's small, but it's the only thing I can do to put ease in your day.

He left before I could ask him his name. I'll never forget what he said. And more important, how he said it. It was so much less about the tip and so much more about his extension of empathy that I remember to this day. I can feel the way my heart lightened, even now. He saw our pain.

I tried to track him down unsuccessfully for months and wrote unreceived letters to let him know how grateful we were for him. As I rewrote my gratitude here, I choked up and felt a surge of warmth in my heart. No lie. Because, here's the deal. When you feel gratitude, the neuroscience shows that not only do you make hormones that help you feel better, but you also produce oxytocin, the *hugging* or *loving* hormone. You want to care for others, and for yourself.

And when you rewrite your experiences of gratitude in detail, as I just did, your brain feels as if it's really happening, all over again. You get double the benefit. Studies show that if you can write about something you're grateful for twenty-one days in a row, you multiply those benefits exponentially. This practice can amplify the effects of therapy alone. You shift your perspective and create what psychologists call a *spiral of Joy.*

Take a Pause

Writing out your gratitude in detail in this way is a practice worth swimming in.

Studies also show that writing a gratitude letter anywhere from one to three times a week for just a few weeks can have effects on well-being at least three months later. Remember, when you write out the details, it's as if your brain is reliving it and cementing it further as something to hold on to. Think about it. Here I am, telling a story about someone's one minute of kindness over a decade ago. Your gratitude transforms from just a good feeling for you inside to a form of goodness in yourself you want to put out into the world. That's the *prosocial* aspect of gratitude that gives it such power.

And there's more. If you read that letter out loud in person or via phone to them, you light up the empathy centers of your brain and quiet the fear. This practice, explained by psychologist Martin Seligman as a gratitude visit, gives the person reading their letter another instant boost in well-being that lasts for at least one month.

This practice can sound self-conscious and a bit uncomfortable. It is. I've done it several times and each time, I feel hesitant right before having to read it: *I'll just give them the letter to read; there should be enough good vibes in that.* I resist it every single time. But then, I'm always glad I went through with it.

Not only because I feel better and the person hearing the letter is touched. There's a benefit that isn't discussed in the studies but one I've repeatedly experienced in real-life practice. When you make the space to do this gratitude visit, you commit time to Joy. You declare that this appreciation, love, and good feelings are worth making time for, no matter how busy your schedules are or how weird this feels. No matter how much you think the other person already knows how thankful you are. (Believe me, they don't.) The hard, the difficult, the unfairness of this life is too easy to swim in. When there is good, when there is deep gratitude, you also deserve to wade in those waters.

PRACTICE: THE GRATITUDE VISIT

Think of someone who you have been grateful for in this world but have not had the chance to tell. Spend some time thinking of specifically why you are grateful, how that person impacted your life, and what it means to you today.

Write them a letter detailing all this. Then make a date to read it to them out loud. You can do this on the phone, in person, or via video call. Seligman encourages you to be purposefully vague about the visit so that the letter is also a surprise for the person you are appreciating, suggesting that the surprise of such gratitude may imprint it even deeper in their learning and memory. If you can't do this, mailing it to them is another option. If you don't know how to get in touch with them, writing the letter will still be powerful for you.

And what if your pain is so thick that you can't think of a story right now of gratitude to repeat or write about? The studies show that even when you listen to others' stories of gratitude, you receive the same effect. In a study where this was done with people listening to Holocaust survivors recount kindness amidst their darkest days, the same areas of the brain light up and calm down.

So, take a moment to think of a story of someone's gratitude you can resonate with. Where does it land in your body? How does it feel? The more you bring that story to your mind and heart, the more ease and speed with which you light up your brain.

WHEN IT FEELS HARD

Say thank you for this pain, for Zubin, for Duchenne muscular dystrophy.

Go to his bed every night and say thank you.

Debbie's assignment was not only infuriating; it felt downright blasphemous. How could she ask a mother to be *thankful* her son was suffering?

But I did it. Through tears, anger, and wanting to give up, night after night, after Zubin was asleep, I did it. It was the first time I had thanked any pain in my life. And it was the the kindling for my revolution.

I'm not superhuman or special. I'm just a mom who was desperate to feel that this life was worth living again.

Saying *thank you* for this pain put me in my body in a revolutionary way. It meant I had to acknowledge this was really happening and here I was, living it. When I turned away from the pain, I was turning away from my son. Saying *thank you* connected me back to Zubin. It taught me to love this life, and him, no matter what.

PRACTICE: A GRATITUDE MEDITATION

Don't start with the hardest thing to thank. Start simple. Use this exercise to build up your gratitude muscle, and when you are ready, you can add in the more difficult things.

1. Sit or lie in a quiet place and take some deep, cleansing breaths.
2. Then, direct the breath to your heart, breathing in and out from that space, imagining that your heart is receiving and offering the breaths.
3. Think of something or someone you are easily grateful for and imagine them in your heart as you inhale and exhale, cycling gratitude back and forth with your breath.
4. Do this for a few minutes if you can, and longer if able. After you express gratitude, notice whether you feel lighter or more ease in your heart and body.
5. This is a nourishing way to start a day and feed your ventral vagus. I do it anytime I need to settle my nervous system, have more focus, or balance challenging thought patterns.

WHEN IT FEELS IMPOSSIBLE

How can we possibly be grateful in the context of oppression, pure evil, or calamitous disaster? Isn't it just false positivity?

I am asked these questions regularly—on my blog, in workshops, from friends. And especially as the world seems to only escalate in tragic and oppressive ways. But my answer persists.

Gratitude takes back your power after the world takes it away.

Don't get me wrong; when life is falling apart right before you, in those acute moments, it's challenging to muster gratitude, and even if you do, it may be simply for waking up for yet another day of this shit or making it through to the next. That you had the profound courage to open your eyes and do it all over again.

But as time passes, a gratitude practice can give you back Justice. Studies map out its effects in the brain, how it lights up the anterior cingulate cortex (ACC) and medial prefrontal cortex (MPFC), areas associated with planning, deep thinking, and, most important, setting context and meaning of an experience. The pain you endure often strips you of one of the most important sources of Joy in life, how you find meaning. Because all evil and disaster can strip you of your humanity.

Gratitude can help you *assign your own new meaning* to it in your MPFC. And the more you do this practice, the brighter and faster the neural circuitry lights up. As little as five minutes of a tool called *gratitude reappraisal or recasting* can decrease the resting state activity of the fear center, the amygdala. It can make you less hypervigilant, creating a new or renewed sense of safety. The way you reframe a traumatic story from the past allows you to feel that safety in the present moment and start the process of healing.

I asked another teacher from my Marjory Stoneman Douglas High School group, Ben, to look back now four years later on that horrific shooting. But not to relive the trauma, to instead gain a new perspective after this space of time and reframe the meaning with this exercise. He told me he now sees that the shooting and his experience of being in the school that day and having to heal have made him *a more sensitive person* and have *more compassion.* He sees how it improved his relationship with his wife because of this growing compassion and his knowing of *what really matters.* He is today, he claims, *more of the person* he would have *wanted to be.*

Like Ben, study participants do not say they are glad the trauma occurred or deny the pain it caused, but by recasting the experience in the light of gratitude, they are able to assign meaning to horrible memories and in a way, redeem them as powerful growth. After the World Trade Center attacks on 9/11, individuals who used gratitude in this way were more likely to experience post-traumatic growth even though challenging emotions remained present as well. This kind of *making meaning out of suffering,* as Viktor Frankl would call it, can nudge you closer on the continuum to Joy than even positive events alone.

Also, my other answer: I simply don't try to find gratitude in all unspeakable times. I let myself feel the anger, frustration, or despair and that is enough. But when I do center the power of gratitude, it's not that *I need to* but because *I deserve to.* I will never make excuses for evil. I cannot find gratitude *in* the injustice, but *I find gratitude for my capacity to see it, to feel the deep grief and sadness I do when confronted with these evils.* If I am feeling all this, I have not lost my humanity. I am still here, feeling the pain, and that gives me hope. I am thankful to walk this journey with others who see it so deeply with me, for fighting together as a community, *for knowing that our power grows as we feel and work together.* And that is all my own truth. As you will have yours.

Gratitude can also be a powerful tool for fighting injustice. In one small study, gratitude practice made individuals more altruistic and likely to care about the state of the world at large. Gratitude is not *putting a positive light* on things; it is allowing universal forces of good to accompany you on this journey through evil and suffering. It is a steadfast tool in Justice work so that you can continue the work of being human in an all-too-often inhumane world.

PRACTICE: GRATITUDE REAPPRAISAL

I offer this exercise because I discussed the power it can have but if the event still lives too strongly in your body, I would highly recommend you do this with a trusted trauma-informed therapist who can guide you through the journey.

You can try this exercise of gratitude recasting with a painful experience. I would suggest trying a simpler one first rather than the most challenging one that comes to mind. Make sure you have some time to yourself to answer and contemplate these questions in writing or dictating as a voice memo if writing is not accessible. First, bring to mind the emotions the experience evokes in you. You do not relive the actual event, but instead what emotions it has left you with; write those down. Once you have done that, take a few breaths (and anytime you need them) and see whether any of the following questions evoke answers for you. If you can, write those answers down, and if you like, share them with someone with whom you feel safe.

Questions:

1. Are you able to find ways to be thankful now for anything that came out of that experience?
2. How has this event benefited you as a person? How have you grown? Were there personal strengths that grew out of your experience?
3. How has the event made you better able to meet the challenges of the future?
4. How has the event put your life in perspective?
5. How has this event helped you appreciate the truly important people and things in your life?

WIDEN YOUR CIRCLE

My younger brother teases me sometimes, calling me *The Gratitude Lady.* After giving a TEDx Talk, writing a blog, and starting a virtual community on the topic, I may not be able to shake that title.

But then I'll also take the liberty, in this last section, of not giving you data from the research labs but instead the ancient science of human experience in one additional exercise I call *Ancestral Circles.*

Because of a daily and ever-present practice, especially through the most difficult times, I feel more connected to and a part of the world around me. Thanking my pain has opened me up to my life, lowered my resistance (remember $S = P \times R$), and cultivated my compassion for others who suffer as well. And over time, all of that has planted me more firmly in connection to my body and this Earth and all the circles of bodies who came before me. I thank my ancestral circles regularly now and with deep reverence. It reminds me that nothing I have done or received is of just my own effort.

Although thanking ancestors is a common ritual in my culture, I did not integrate it fully until weaving a gratitude practice into my life more firmly. It settles my body, most likely stimulating that ventral vagal pathway in the most ancient of ways. I don't have a randomized study to tell you it works. But I'm not waiting for one.

PRACTICE: ANCESTRAL CIRCLES

You can try this exercise when you are feeling alone, isolated in your suffering, or as well when you are feeling Joyful and want to express gratitude for that moment. Call on the ancestors you need most in any moment, depending on what you are experiencing. This is a practice done in a multitude of cultures around the world in a multitude of ways. This exercise is not the only way, just one example.

1. Find a quiet place in your home. I sit at an altar I have created, but you can choose any spot you find supportive. An ancestral altar can often include pictures, objects that remind you of your ancestors or that come directly from them, or items from

nature, just to name a few. Some are called to do an offering to their ancestors before even starting. This will depend on your cultural rituals or ones you begin to cultivate. For me, it's incense. For some, it's tobacco or other plants, food, or the use of sound. This is unique to you.

2. After you do this, close your eyes and make an intention. A wish for what you need. Say it out loud or think on it. I will give you an example. If I am feeling stuck in fear for my son's future, I might state a wish for comfort or hope.
3. Then, I take a few breaths and watch the inhale and exhale wherever that is easiest—as it enters my nose or mouth or the back of my throat, or as it comes out.
4. Once I have taken at least three to five breaths, I imagine myself sitting in a safe space. One where I am in the middle and ancestors appear in a circle around me. One by one. In this case, maybe it's ancestors who have also feared for their lives or someone they love, ones who have an understanding of how my heart trembles.
5. You do not even need to know who they are, just that they are safe, loving beings.
6. As they sit around you, they send you their love, strength, and blessings. You inhale these and exhale gratitude to the circle around you. Over and over.
7. Continue in this way for as long as you like, but try to do it for five to ten minutes minimum if you can. If distractions arise or thoughts interfere, that is okay. Let them float to the side, and bring your attention back to the breath and then the circle around you.

8. Maybe you set a bell timer on your phone or just end when you feel ready. Notice whether your heart or body feels different. Or whether you learned a message to keep close to your heart. Come back to this meditation as often as you like for a few minutes or more.

CHAPTER 12

It's Not Forgiveness, It's Grace

FORGET FORGIVENESS

I am so tired of forgiveness. My body bristles every time I think about it. I know the science. I know it heals. But it also needs to fit my revolution. I am tired of being asked to do work for *someone else's* wrongs. I've worked enough to just be here and start each day.

I often can't forgive the unfairness in my life and I sure as hell can't forgive evil, but I can give myself the grace to live in this world and prosper despite all that.

Grace comes from the Latin *gratus*, "thankful." It is a direct descendant of being grateful.

When I think of *giving grace*, I think of it as a powerful action, of giving space to all that needs to be here so that it can flow into what it needs to be. Joy, and you, need space to thrive.

If I give myself grace, I am softening to myself and whatever wrongs or hurts I may have caused to others or myself.

If I give my anger or pain grace, I am accepting the beauty of myself no matter how I stand in this moment.

If I give someone grace for a wrong imposed on me, I am accepting that they, too, are human—not the kind I need around me, but a human nonetheless. And in that space I have created, I can see that we both have flaws without excusing the ways theirs have hurt me. And they can go do their own work while I do mine.

This may sound like forgiveness to you. I think in a way, it is similar. And I suspect then that the science of forgiveness also applies to grace, so I will take the liberty of using it. There is a big difference to me, though, in which action feels most revolutionary.

Forgiveness is all about what the world is asking of you.

Grace is what you are asking back from the world.

After Zubin was born, before all the horrible news about DMD, I had the kind of postpartum depression you read about in books or see in the movies, the kind that my husband described as *I wasn't sure if you were ever coming back to us.* And I can say for sure now that it was made much worse by trying to also live my regular life, mother my other son, doctor and take overnight calls, teach and create new programs, all of it while also keeping this shame-ridden truth to myself. That when I went home at night, I didn't want to be a mother to this child or even, frankly, be here. Less than a handful of people in my life knew this truth. And even as I write this, I'm taking deep breaths to settle my nervous system and body because all painful memories still attach to tense places that recoil when vulnerability emerges.

I don't recommend to anyone to hide this kind of truth. Even though I eventually sought help, keeping it inside nearly killed me. We can convince ourselves that the challenge is a failing of our own, but our most tender mental health ailments are like any condition that needs external support. You need teams around you, medical and social, for support and to help just get the mundane tasks of life done.

My depression lasted in its darkest iteration for almost a year, but even after I thought it was *better*, I did not realize that it was taking up so much space within me that I could not feel the depths of Joy or pain the way I used to. Most likely, my dorsal vagus had kicked in to get me through this pain. In essence, I had numbed.

Over a year and a half after Zubin's birth I was in a training to do the trauma work I do now in small groups. I was doing a body scan (the way I described in Chapter 9), but this time, the result was not so instantly blissful.

We were instructed to visit parts of our body and listen for messages. When we were in our pelvis, I had a clear image of my uterus and the pull to stay there was so strong that as the instructions guided us up to our abdomen and chest, I stayed behind. And I heard loud and clear, *Forgive me. Forgive me.*

I started crying and the tears would not stop. In that instant, I knew that even though my mood had stabilized and I had started mothering again, I had not forgiven myself for what felt like the most *shameful* act of abandoning my son by not loving him fully. And so, I stayed and breathed deeply. Listening over and over, *Forgive me, forgive me.* Until I started to trust that it spoke truth I needed to hear.

I went to my uterus in my own meditation for weeks on end after this. I tried to offer forgiveness as it had asked but found this challenging, as I had already been softening to the truth that my depression had not been a failing that *needed* forgiving but instead a part of my humanness that *deserved* grace. Soft, tender grace for being human. For being desperately sad and disconnected. For feeling such pain and for the pain it caused my family.

Make no mistake: grace is a soft space, but it is also fiercely powerful.

Take a Pause

What is it you may deserve grace for? Think of a time when you have imposed superhuman expectations on yourself. Can you realize you were only human? A human who failed, hurt someone, or merely suffered from a human condition. Where can you soften and give yourself grace? It is a revolutionary act that you can do for yourself when the world has not given you enough.

FORGET THE HOOK

If you've been wronged, you have the right to your anger. I know that deep in my bones.

Your anger started as an act of self-love, truly. It was your brain and heart's way of keeping some illusion of control over this wrong. *If I just stay mad at this person or system, the injustice is real.* And that anger is needed to move to action, in most cases.

If you eventually soften to the anger, by giving it grace and allowing it to be, you are not asking it to change or diminish. You merely get curious about your anger, like an unknown guest.

And then you can see more clearly whether there are any ways the emotion could also be diminishing you. Chronic, unrelenting anger, for instance, keeps you in a stressed-out, fight-or-flight mode. Your nervous system evaluates this landscape as meaning you are in constant battle. Which weakens your immune and cardiovascular systems and makes you *more* depressed and anxious. Now the perpetrator is really winning.

Giving grace to a person doesn't absolve anyone of a wrong. It doesn't mean you've let them off the hook, as the saying goes. Grace is about liberating yourself and acquiring more space and ease.

When you offer grace to yourself or the world, *you* finally win. Your stress hormones go down, you feel less depression and anxiety, your immune system fights infections, you sleep more soundly, your blood pressure decreases, your heart works better. And better yet, it isn't good for you just while you do it. Even six months after the practice, benefits—including increased compassion and optimism—are present.

Now, I won't lie. This is a process. You can't fake this shit. Your body knows the difference. You can't just say *I offer grace* and get all the benefits. You have to really feel it. But here's the deal: The more you feel it, the more you develop compassion for yourself and even others. And you already know how good that is for you.

A few disclaimers:

Grace doesn't mean you always forget. This hurt might always be with you. But it won't hold you in a vice grip the same way. As you soften your body, your hold on the pain eases as well.

Let go of expectations for others. This is your grace to give. You don't even have to share it out loud. Some people honestly do not respond in a healing way and you don't need that. Make this about you, not them.

Grace doesn't mean you need to seek reconciliation. In fact, many times that's not the safest thing to do.

And the biggest question I get: *What if I just cannot offer grace?* Then, it's a good time for self-compassion, my love. Some hurts are just so big and hard that you aren't ready to soften, maybe ever. The best you can do is try, and if it doesn't feel right or welcome, move on. Truly. There are many steps to Joy and those steps may even clear a path for grace at a later time. Don't beat yourself up over this. Life has already done that; this is a road map to a gentler way of being. Move lightly on.

How slow or fast you want to take it, and stopping anytime you need to, is all up to you. This is about being loving with yourself when the world has neglected to do so. And here's a secret: If you start with the easier things—the person who cut you off in traffic today—you can work up. Don't start with the person you've most resented your whole life. You need to build up that muscle. Trust me. This is a *practice*; proceed with gentle care.

Here are some approaches you can consider:

Decide someone or something deserves your grace. Keep that intention real and close when you start the process, whenever that is. Your own time, in your own way.

Always include yourself in the practice. Even if you weren't the one who perpetuated the wrong, somewhere, somehow along the way, you might link the injustice to your own worth. You deserve not to harden to life the way the suffering has hardened you.

Practice it over and over until you deeply feel the release. There is no deadline. Use your favorite prayer, meditation, or reflection, or work with a trusted guide or therapist. You'll know the release when your body feels lighter and, yet, stronger.

Become an observer in the practice. This helps to cultivate compassion for the person or world, not because they deserve it, but because doing so will open and soften *your* heart, to yourself and your own anger. Researchers describe a practice called psychological distancing that can help you *step back and... reflect on the course of action instead of being dominated by immediate stimulation* to your nervous system. Two tangible ways to create this space are explained in the practices at the end of the section. Studies show it helps you diffuse the emotional charge and regulate your nervous system, changes that can begin as fast as just a few seconds.

Take a Pause

I think of distancing techniques not as cognitive hacks that are presented in the wellness world, but rather as elegant tools of Justice. You are creating safety within yourself so that you can do the work you need for liberation. If you see a situation as a threat, you go into stress mode, but if you see the exact same situation as a challenge, you think, feel, and perform better. Distancing from the harm allows you to see your capacity for change.

And here's the biggest secret: Even if you feel that you never get there, the mere consideration of giving grace unlocks your body's deep entanglement in anger, resentment, and fear along the way. One study showed that even thinking about giving an offender grace improved cardiovascular and nervous systems. The act of *trying* means you're winning this fight for Justice because your grace is doing more for yourself than the world is doing for you.

PRACTICE: PSYCHOLOGICAL DISTANCING

These two techniques may give you the distance you need to do the work.

1. One is to create space between you and the giving of the grace. Notice when you reflect on giving grace for a situation or person: What happens in your body? Are you constricted or tense? Where? Just notice. Take a few breaths and now notice what happens if you reflect on the same situation, but with distance by imagining it as a movie playing out in front of you. Notice how your body feels when you do this instead of imagining yourself immersed in it.

   Literally imagine you are watching yourself do this, like a movie. It makes sense that distance can diffuse the emotional charge a bit by taking you out of your body for a moment to observing your body, as if going from first- to third-person perspective. You see the situation more in the way you would if you were helping a friend. And in fact, just as you would talk to that friend, using your own name as you talk yourself through this can amplify the power of this distancing.

2. Or you can create space with time by picturing your future self looking back on this moment and imagining how they would advise your current self or view the situation. When you create this *temporal space*, as it is called, you might be less focused on the immediate, concrete aspects of the dilemma of grace and instead see it in a broader context of how it might fit into your life as a whole.

   You can make this type of distancing practical by writing a letter to yourself from your future self. What would you, five or ten years from now, say to yourself about this situation? What wisdom or guidance would you offer? What might you have learned about grace or this specific situation in the future? Imagine if you give grace now. What might this future self thank you for?

WRITE YOUR OWN STORY

Ben, who I mentioned earlier, was one of my favorites in that July 2018 small group. The way he choked up when he talked about his work touched me deeply. When Ben shared with the group the intense fear he felt to walk back into the school, his suffering was palpable. His voice quivered as he explained the horrors of how that afternoon in February unfolded. In an instant, the place he felt most at home in, outside his own, had become a bloodbath and he was absolutely sure he could not feel safe again.

When I think of how one could even ask Ben to forgive the shooter, I feel enraged *for* him. But Ben's reappraisal years later taught me not only about gratitude, but an even more powerful lesson on grace: *It (the trauma) rearranged what is important to me and what should be appreciated. Connections have become much more important. I've gained compassion and understanding that I will never be able to unlearn.*

Ben had made space for grace, not for the shooter per se, but for how the shooting had changed him. When we *reappraise* the stories of the wrongs or tragedy, we move toward greater Joy and better health. Ruminating keeps us in a tight, toxic grip while rewriting the narrative gives us power. The practice of reappraising also gives the story, itself, grace: that it has a different meaning than we or the world assigned it to begin with. I love that because it means that when we take ownership and power back, our body recognizes this as healing. And this is Justice.

I want to be clear. This is not *putting things in a positive light or looking on the bright side.* The power in this rewriting of the story is in *owning the most human parts of yourself and this world.* That is the Justice here. It's in seeing your deep, inner well of goodness that is indestructible regardless of what happened or who wronged you. This powerful act of giving grace is about recognizing we all have the capacity to be wronged—and to wrong others as well. It is seeing all of us as broken and whole in our brokenness.

If you choose to try this work, do it gently, give yourself time, pause often, and seek the support of your most trusted people. If you choose not to enter, give yourself grace that this feels too hard to do right now, and maybe ever. Go back to another tool and focus there. No one way is more right or measures your value or capacity more than another. We all find our Justice path somewhere that is right for us. Walk yours with power and grace.

PRACTICE: GIVING YOURSELF GRACE

The work of giving grace can take time and may not even be what you want right now. You can always give yourself grace, no matter what, and I would encourage you to start the practice there.

1. Remember to try something small at first. Take baby steps. This is not simple.
2. Before you start, think of the situation for which you are giving yourself grace, either for something you or someone else blames you for, a way you have disappointed yourself, or for not wanting to or being able to give grace in a challenging situation.
3. Get in a comfortable position and take at least three to five deep breaths with a slower exhale each time. Creating space in your body with breath is important and you want to engage your sense of safety. Close your eyes if able or keep them on a soft gaze down or ahead.
4. Imagine yourself sitting across from you in a chair. That self can be any age you like.
5. Send that self love and compassion for showing up here today. Take a few deep breaths together.
6. Imagine saying one or more of the following phrases: "I give you grace for any way I have disappointed or wronged you. I give you grace because you are human. I give you grace

because you deserve that Justice." (You, of course, make the phrases right for you.)

7. If able, repeat this or your own set of phrases three times. Take three more deep breaths together.
8. If doing this is challenging and you would rather write, you can imagine you are writing yourself a letter and write those phrases or anything else that comes with them in the letter. You can also ask someone to mail you the sealed letter at a later time.

PART III

RECLAIM YOUR JOY

CHAPTER 13

In Your Body

Do you remember the moment you learned to ride a bike? Imagine your body wavering in fearful imbalance back and forth on a two-wheeled vehicle, one foot tenuously touching the ground on either side to give you a sense of safety. Or the moment you learned to read? Recall your mind and body tensing in stringent concentration to piece together unintelligible letters on a page into patterns that made sense. In either example, hearing in your mind, *I will never be able to do this.* Even sometimes falling on the ground and thinking, *I am tired of getting hurt* or slamming the book, wondering, *Why does this seem so easy for everyone else?* But then in a magical moment that seems to emerge both spontaneously and as the sum of all your diligent effort, both of your feet rest on the pedals, miraculously at the same time, and incredibly, the bike propels forward, or the words merge into a way that you now see the world more clearly, both taking you on a freedom ride of sorts, and you feel your mind and body hovering in a blissful balance. You go from overthinking the mechanics of *how* to your body knowing and trusting that it *can* and never being able to unknow this magic from that moment on. It took practice, lots of practice, and trust, so much trust, but now it is part of you. And such will be the integration of Joy in your body. Joy is a part of you that has always been present, but now it is allowed to emerge through that tender mingling of practice and faith.

CHAPTER 14

In Awe

It was –38 degrees Celsius (which doesn't even need conversion in my Fahrenheit-centric world to know it's too cold!) and I was outside. That in and of itself was a feat of heroism for this warm-sun-loving Desi girl. But the cold was the last thing on my mind. I was, instead, transfixed. The vast, ink-black, star-studded sky stretched farther above me than I had ever known it could. Lights of iridescent green had started dancing, literally undulating, across the sky, turning hues, even adding pinks. I felt pure awe. That a performance like this could exist. That I could be standing on the Earth viewing it. My small self in a vast, vast universe. I watched it for hours, I was told. But time had stood still for me in that moment. All I knew was that there was something greater than anything I understood or had tried to ever reason through. As I looked down at Zubin, he locked eyes with me. *Do you think these lights will heal us, Mama?*

The scientific explanation of the northern lights is that gaseous particles from the Earth's atmosphere collide with charged particles from the sun. But collision sounded too violent to me as I viewed this magical sky. Indigenous peoples across the Arctic lands had stared for centuries at this miracle and trusted their own intuitive wisdom to make sense of what danced before them. I loved the belief that these lights were the dancing spirits of lost loved ones, including beloved sled dogs, on their way to the afterworld. But the science and stories all fell to the side of the truth I felt in my body in that moment. The bite of the cold air on my face, the sight of the colorful lights moving across the large expanse of black sky, the hollow sounds of nighttime silence. I knew this experience was worth zooming into, immersing in as fully as possible. This moment of awe reminded me that holding Joy right now, right here, could also help me hold the swirl of emotions in my heart and reminded me of my profound capacity to love, not only my children, but myself as a mother. That this vast universe could hold so much, even all my doubt, grief, and fear.

The science shows that moments of awe can have a prosocial result, the desire to step forward and care for the collective. An interesting and so artfully simple study with Berkeley students showed that even after just a minute in the middle of the campus's towering eucalyptus tree grove versus looking at a school building, students were more likely to show generosity or aid to a stranger. Even fleeting experiences of awe can have an impact on how we feel about others. I think again of our ancestors who stood and wondered at sights like those lights. Possibly, their practice of awe connected them, too, to something greater and encouraged their focus to tend to one another.

Leading researchers on awe offer their definitions to guide us in recognizing this practice in ourselves. Let them sink in for a moment.

Awe is being amazed and astonished by the vastness of something. —Dacher Keltner

Awe distorts time perception by making it stand still. —Melanie Rudd

Once we have seen past ourselves, we can be open to what the world and others offer. —Jennifer Stellar

If I could have dinner with them, I would add that the mere act of having awe for something else eventually translates into you having awe for yourself: if you are able to behold the wonder, then you, too, must be a part of it.

Seek moments of awe as often as you can, from great, majestic moments to the seemingly mundane, and then intentionally linger in them. I think of them as Joy boosters. It's not just me; the literature describes how moments of awe lower inflammation, and increase well-being and even your humility. The word *humility* is rooted in the Latin word *humus*, meaning "soil" or "ground." Awe returns you to the soil of who you are.

It's easy to see it in the most clichéd of things—flowers, butterflies, a sunset. But can you find it in the mundane of your unique day-to-day life? I have to remind myself not to brush off Zubin's now numerous daily *I love you*'s or the way I turn on the faucet and water just comes right out, but both are wondrous in their own right. Where are you brushing off awe? This world is treacherous and, at the same time, not. You deserve to bask in that power.

Take a Pause

Let this sink in. The critical piece here is not only that the world can be awe-inspiring but that *you deserve* to feel it all. Each time you take in a moment of wonder, I think of it as inhaling your life force (remember that the word *breath* literally means this in some traditions). You begin to look for moments of awe not only to feel better but to feel fully alive.

Science has now found that having moments such as this, not only connect us to something greater but also regulate and balance our autonomic nervous system in powerful ways. Sophisticated brain imaging, such as fMRI, shows that awe is actually *felt* by our nervous system in similar ways to deep prayer or meditation.

In an experience of awe, a different part of your brain, the parietal lobe, the area associated with orienting yourself in this physical world, also shuts down. When those lines are blurred, you experience a sensation of oneness and connectedness. You feel more aligned with humanity instead of persecuted by it. I felt this poignancy when I read about the *overview effect*, a cognitive change that has been seen in astronauts who leave the Earth and view it from space, experiencing what may be the most ultimate definition of *vast* I can think of. So big and wondrous it is that astronauts have likened that now iconic view of the blue-marbled Earth to being what *God must see*.

When you get this wider perspective, the awe you feel can stimulate all those good juice prosocial hormones like dopamine, making you want to do this more; serotonin, making you feel good in the moment; and oxytocin, making you want to connect. German astronaut Sigmund Jähn shared: *Only when I saw it (Earth) from space, in all its ineffable beauty and fragility, did I realize that humankind's most urgent task is to cherish and preserve it for future generations.* Awe makes you want to work for the collective.

Awe also takes you out of your ruminating mind by turning off the default mode network. When I was staring at those northern lights dancing in the sky, all I knew was that there was something wondrous happening before me, and I was somehow an important part of it. Time stood still and I, in it. For those moments, the chatter of my regretful mind fell to the side.

A study of older individuals, between the ages of sixty and ninety, showed that a simple enough practice called an *awe walk* could not only improve their ability to find awe over time but their capacity for gratitude and compassion as well. They reported an increasingly *smaller sense of self* in the vastness of the world around them. A paradox of sorts: they felt smaller and yet more a part of the bigger world surrounding them.

Take a Pause

In the study, the walk, only fifteen minutes, once weekly for eight weeks, feels like a doable practice. I also love that participants walked through *both* cities and nature landscapes, recognizing that not everyone has safe green spaces. This practice is so simple and I, think, modifiable: you can roll on a wheelchair or sit in a new place outside each time and notice the world passing by you, what I would call an *awe roll* or an *awe watch*. Make this journey work for you.

Integrating a practice of Joy unlocks your capacity for wonder and awe for the life in front of you, especially the most mundane parts. You find the wonder in the ordinary and the ordinary becomes more wondrous. And you are changed because of it. You are not the same, nor do you want to be.

PRACTICE: AWE WALK/ROLL/WATCH

Think about integrating this awe practice into your life once a week. Schedule it in your calendar. Make a commitment to yourself that this is what you deserve. You can do it indoors or outdoors, in a city or the countryside. Novelty helps so you can choose different spaces from time to time if able. And like I mentioned in the preceding Take a Pause—roll, walk, or even sit, and most important, notice.

1. Try not to use your phone or listen to anything during the walk. If you want to take a picture of your piece of awe you find, that is okay, to share with someone or document for yourself.
2. In the study I mentioned, they had the individuals take a selfie before and after the walk each time. And they found those on the awe walks had bigger smiles as the study progressed, and also within the picture itself, they increasingly focused on the scene around them and less on themselves, making

themselves physically a smaller part of the pictures as the study went on.

3. Look for pieces of awe in the vastness of the scene—a piece of architecture, the sky, large pieces of art in a museum, large trees—as well as those that are smaller and ask of you a narrower focus, such as flowers, animals, or insects.
4. Do this once weekly for one to two months and notice, if you can, whether the practice gets easier, whether it makes you feel different either during or after you do it. Or whether you feel more awe in your daily life. Share what you notice with someone or in a journal and look back over it.

CHAPTER 15

In Beauty

Some moments of awe overlap with our experience of beauty in this world, whether it be that of art, nature, or music. But I would argue that beauty is worth exploring on its own as both a Joy booster and as a reinoculation against the pain of this world. Science quantifies beauty by a wonderful term, an *aesthetic chill*, that feeling you get when the hair on your arms literally stands up in attention, when a goose bump chill signals to you that something is worth stopping for. Your Joy practices of acceptance, love, gratitude, hope, and grace are what allow you to see beauty more clearly, not just the pain. When you notice this beauty, you see the world more clearly—this dance of being human in an imperfect world, accepting and allowing like an inhale and exhale. You harness hope in the recognition that despite all the terror and deceit, the world cannot be diminished; it persists in its beauty as well. And noticing it becomes a rhythm so natural that it eventually happens daily without your consciously trying.

Scientists have studied the impact of finding beauty on our brain. When you appreciate beauty, your brain lights up its reward centers, increasing its dopamine levels, making you want to seek out even more. This is one way to create an upward spiral of Joy in your brain as opposed to the downward one that can occur when you live only in fear or worry. And more important, it is a spiral *you* can create, from your own power, to give your body what it deserves, Joy. This is your Justice, every day.

In scientific literature, beauty is often quantified as an *openness to experience*. This gives researchers a way to study who is *open* to beauty and who is closed to it. Those higher on the openness scale have less chance of dying from cardiac death.

Take a Pause

Let that sink in. People who are more open to beauty have a healthier heart.

Not only that, but brain scans show that these individuals have turned down their default mode network. Researchers postulate that being open to beauty may ultimately *serve a stress inoculation function* due to the combination of *enlarged cognition and peak emotions*. In plain speak, beauty makes you think differently about the world because you learn to feel something different in your body.

PRACTICE: YOUR OWN BEAUTY WATCH

What is your concept of beauty? And how do you take it in? By observation, drawing, writing, taking a picture? What if you started a beauty journal? It does not have to be so regimented as a daily requirement. Just a place where you document beauty because it deserves your attention.

A photo, a few lines describing it, a sketch, a poem or quote that inspires you, or a photo of any art. You keep it in one place so you can look at it on days when beauty is more obscure, when your mind is clouded and needs a little reminder.

It could be a physical journal, a folder on your computer, an old-fashioned scrapbook, or even a voice recorder app on your phone.

CHAPTER 16

In Faith

In 1662, *Atocha*, a Spanish ship, sank in a hurricane 35 miles from Key West with a treasure trove of over $130 million in gems. The gems were not recovered until 1985 by a salvage team. This, in and of itself, is not the most spectacular part of the story when you also learn what else was salvaged over 365 years from the incident. Seeds. Seeds of various kinds, grapes, apricots, and more, which lay more than 55 feet under the surface. Seeds that by all purposes should have been dead. But instead, after recovery, they sprouted. Preserved under heavy planks and mud under the sea, they then grew. I tell you this, not to go into a long discourse of how this could be possible biologically (apparently there is still debate on how they survived because it is so miraculous), but instead to marvel at the power of a seed.

The potential of what lies in a seed mirrors the potential of what lies in you, always. No matter how deeply buried, under the muck of suffering, it exists. But when you suffer, you lose sight of the seeds. The practice of Joy untangles not only the potential of what you have ready to germinate but, as well, even the sheer faith that seeds are waiting to be uncovered. Joy nurtures faith in this world and in yourself.

When Zubin was diagnosed, so many dreams were shattered for me. Dreams of a child growing up and running in the yard, playing sports or instruments, going to college, or starting his own family. Dreams of our intact family, not one disrupted by countless medical visits, medical scares, and caregiving. These dreams were replaced only by fears until I learned to nurture myself with Joy. Joy in and of itself felt like an internal revolution because it felt like the most unattainable thing then, even more than a cure.

I still remember when Zubin had the gift of speeding down a snowy mountain in a sit-ski. When he reached the bottom, after feeling so free, fast, and alive, we all had tears in our eyes, including his adaptive guide. I looked blurrily at Steve and said what has become a mantra for us both: *There is always more than one way to come down a mountain.*

It is still true that I can say Zubin shattered so many dreams. But what I now add is that I had no idea the dreams I would piece back together would be bigger than anything I had conceived of as possible. That my heart would have the capacity to hold more, more pain than I had ever known but also more Joy. That I would expand beyond my limited understanding of what a *good and worthy* life is. And that I could cultivate faith in the darkest of times, no matter what.

What you don't know about that moment with the northern lights was that it came at the end of a week when Zubin broke his leg in the middle of nowhere, a life-threatening event in a boy with DMD due to a potential catastrophic complication. I had regressed into a dark spiral of guilt and regret, doubting my capacity to mother him or live this life. When Zubin asked whether those lights could heal, I teared up and nodded yes, because the lights were reflecting back our own capacity to illuminate deep darkness. That Arctic sky was as vast as if looking out at an ocean from an island and imagining the next piece of land could never be seen. It was that wide, all-encompassing, and even intimidating. But on that night, the lights, which had been evasive to us every evening prior, reminded me of my Justice. I was still standing, enduring, and staying present just like those dancing lights had for millennia. I could still feel awe, see their beauty, and have faith that this life was not only *for* me, but I was here *for my life*. Because when you show up to find faith, and Joy, despite the pain, you are as alive as you will ever feel.

Take a Pause

When your faith that Joy is yours to have falters, it is helpful to go back to your deeper why or your own truth. What is it? Is it still true or has it changed? How can you reinforce it for yourself? Through movement, breath, or writing, for example. Remember your truth is yours to have, yours to alter, and always there for you.

CHAPTER 17

In Fear

Joy does not dissolve all fear. A life without fear is impossible and, I would challenge, not useful. Fear is a protective mechanism that has helped our species survive. And it is also an important signal you need to listen to, often uncovering your deepest intuition about potential harm. Especially if you are in a vulnerable community, it is an important messenger: take heed and use it to gain clarity for action. But when it is in overdrive, disrupts your ability to function, or gives you a false signal of danger, it ceases to serve you.

The practice of Joy expands your capacity to hold fear without its dysfunction. So that it can be an important companion, a powerful messenger that either something in the environment is amiss or something *within you* is out of balance.

And possibly the best way to learn what your fear needs you to know is the use of your breath. Holding your breath will amplify fear and distort its messages. So, let your breath flow into the fear to give it movement, to get it unstuck. Move and shake your body, if able, to let it flow. Tune in to which kind of fear it is, of which there are usually three broad types.

The kind of fear that is present in a real threat will remain, but you will have more capacity to know what to do next. *Listen well.*

The fear of only a perceived threat may dissipate or will gain needed clarity. *You are okay. You can do this.*

And then there is the magical third kind of fear that may be left—the one you feel when your heart quivers in excitement, knowing you are at the precipice of your truth, even though it feels uncomfortable in your body. *This discomfort is a growing pain; all change is hard.*

Joy sustains the faith that your fear can serve its purpose if you continue to meet it in your body and breathe into it, both physically and metaphorically. A more difficult task to say than do, yet remember it is a challenge of being human, to get comfortable in your discomfort.

Accept the fear in the present moment with curiosity.

Give it gratitude for being here, that it may have a purpose yet unseen.

Love it as a tender, deserving part of you.

Use your breath to ride it like the crest of a wave until it softens or dissipates.

Give yourself grace for any shame, doubt, or resistance.

Give your fear the respect it deserves *and* do not allow it to own you at the same time.

PRACTICE: TONGLEN MEDITATION

This practice is not an easy one. If you are feeling fear or dread that is getting stuck even after using breath, the tools from Part 2, or work with a therapist, consider adding this ancient Buddhist exercise. It elegantly works with compassion and suffering in a way that reminds us we are all human and struggle with the world at large. You can do this practice anytime, even on the spot if you see someone suffering and that causes fear in you. The goal is not to erase fear but to be more comfortable sitting with it.

1. First attend to your breath, just noticing it as it goes in and out.
2. Then, imagine the pain at hand. Maybe it's the pain of someone you love or of a community in the world that has stirred fear for you. Maybe it's your own pain, in this case, possibly your own fear. Imagine it as a dark, inky, smokelike substance in front of you.
3. On your inhale, breathe it into your heart. It may feel uncomfortable to do so. Go slow and be tender. If it's too much, you can stop again and try another time.
4. Imagine it radiating through your heart to your whole body as if you are taking in this pain fully.
5. When you exhale, imagine you are letting out a bright light of compassion or a clearing of the smoke. Imagine it radiating from your whole body and heart. Repeat this over and over, inhaling the smoke and breathing out the lightness and cleared air.
6. Make the inhales and exhales bigger as you are able. Taking more in and also releasing more each time.
7. As you do this, imagine breathing out the clearing and lightness for all who share this pain. Imagine the expansive world of those who suffer just the same.
8. Grow the breath as you grow your capacity to feel the suffering, but also the compassion that the lightness brings.

9. Do this for five to ten minutes, or as long or short that feels right to you.
10. Over time, this practice can increase your compassion for yourself and others but also get you more comfortable with challenging emotions like fear. Instead of resisting them, you literally take more of it in.
11. As I said, it can also be done on the spot as you get more agile with the exercise. So that if you see someone suffering, you can inhale in fear and darkness and breathe out light and compassion.

CHAPTER 18

In *Your* Purpose

You deserve to know *your purpose*, but in your way.

Yes, studies show that people with a sense of purpose sleep better, have a stronger immune system, secrete less stress hormones, and even live longer. So, that may explain why you hear the wellness world wax on about how to discover yours, but is that an equitable ask? One of the most common psychological scales for assessing a sense of purpose implies its levels of privilege, including such statements as:

In general, I feel I am in charge of the situation in which I live.

I sometimes feel as if I've done all there is to do in life.

One of the meanings of purpose that you will find in the dictionary includes a *goal* or *intention*. And that has been co-opted by our capitalist doer society as a way of proving your worth or your way of *giving back* to the world. In fact, another item on the scale asks about the degree to which others would say you are a giving person and willing to share time with others. If you have the capacity to serve others, that's wonderful and welcome. But if you don't because you're working too hard trying to financially or emotionally survive, how would you fare on this scale?

Researchers describe a sense of purpose as a kind of psychological homeostasis that allows an individual to navigate daily stress with the most ease possible. And those who face the most adversity may feel a strong sense of purpose if they are able to assign meaning to this challenge. But inherent in the assessment of purpose as a marker of well-being is an inequitable distribution of the capacity to qualify. It's time for a reframe.

Purpose is not a one-and-done nirvana plan. Your purpose today can look very different than tomorrow. Today may be survival, tomorrow resistance. And the next day, rest. Who knows? Only you, that's who. Your purpose no matter what, in any given moment, can be to just exist in this torn-up, exhausting world. That you are still here, reading this book, contemplating a better day. You get to decide, but you also do not need to be constrained by an archaic view of purpose that implies you have to already be feeling moments of peace along the way. No, instead, finding purpose right here, in this very moment, can be your exact path to that ease.

If you've been in bed for the last year, unable to engage with life, or completely disconnected, your purpose is your first step tomorrow, even if one teensy one forward. If you've been dreaming of being Joyful but instead are having something close to the proverbial midlife crisis, your purpose may be first to recognize everything around you, and then either thank it for being beautiful or for being so dreadful that it moved you to want change. Thank every last bit of it. See it all as purpose. It's exactly what will propel you to clarity. It's what will carry you to Joy.

Your purpose can be to exist for meaning greater than yourself. For your ancestors who toiled before you, for your community who walks alongside you, for those yet to come and walk in your footsteps. Or to exist simply because you can. Because you are worthy of that. Purpose is not a privilege; it's your right.

Take a Pause

What if your wounds aren't all meant to heal right away? I know that may be a downright blasphemous thing for a physician to say. But none of us can fix everything. Sometimes your purpose may be to merely *be with* and listen to your pain. No, you don't deserve pain or hurt, ever. And at the same time, I cannot remove the inexorable truth that to hurt is to be human. No matter the source, some wounds may be too big to heal right now. The mere fact that they continue to seep and bleed may mean that they are here to guide you back to yourself.

If you don't feel ready to send love to your life or wounds, then it's also a tender time to call back in compassion and grace. You don't have to feel good about anything in anyone else's time. You are not broken. Not feeling purposefully driven in the way the world defines it does not detract from who you are. Your spiritual practice is yours to design. Spend some moments back in the sections on compassion and grace and remember that you are the architect of your Joy practice. Your practice right now, today, can be to love who you are even if where you stand feels hard. Love yourself for standing anyway. And do that *with purpose.*

CHAPTER 19

In *Your* Resilience

Resilience is what the world asks of you when you weather challenge, but your Justice is in how you choose to answer that.

You suffer and yet are asked to then feel good.

You thrive and yet are asked to then do more.

Have you stopped to think that maybe, just maybe, some who are deemed the most *resilient* have disconnected so much from their body's messages because of trauma or hardship that the only way they know to meet a challenge is to push even harder? And then, they are thought to be the *strongest* when in fact they are further weakening their nervous systems. This was my experience in medical training and then for two-plus decades working with resident physicians. In medicine, we often measure ourselves and our peers by who is not *doing well* or who is *having a hard time* if they need a break or professional help. But maybe they are the ones who are fully in their body to feel the pain and know they need to do something different from *pushing through*.

A study in first-year resident physicians was the first of its kind to measure telomere length before and after an intense period of shared challenge. Telomeres are the caps on DNA that keep them from unraveling. Think of them as the plastic ends to your shoelaces that prevent fraying. Science has shown that they get shorter with stressors and oppression and damage our DNA, literally aging you more rapidly. In this study, the residents had changes in their telomeres so marked that they aged six times faster than their peers! And the more hours they worked, the bigger the changes.

Their so-called resilience was literally killing them. I shudder to think of how I have wielded this version of resilience, given to me in overt and implicit ways, against myself and others (and so, I ask for grace), and now I seek to reclaim a liberated meaning. I will add my own theory to the study's finding that the residents were not only aging themselves but imprinting even deeper the habit of disconnecting from their body's messages. And mind you, this is not their fault, but instead one of the medical training system at large that deems their worthiness on this *strength*.

Take a Pause

Ask yourself whether how you are meeting a challenge is truly the best way for you. Yes, life does not always provide the simplest way to advocate for what you need. There are financial, societal, and cultural pressures that make taking rest, for example, unacceptable or impossible. But are there ways you can push back at all on these pressures? And in what ways can you be gentle and loving with yourself in listening to your body?

After twenty years of delivering babies, I went to my director and asked to be taken off Obstetrics call. It was one of my most challenging professional transitions. Delivering babies was one of my biggest Joys (but also biggest stressors). I was now giving that up and, moreover, I risked my job by asking for what I needed. Care for Zubin, especially overnight care, had become its own form of night call on top of everything else my mothering and job demanded of me. He said yes but then called me in only days later to say that my group had told him it *was not fair* and to rethink my ask. I began to doubt myself, but I persisted. I told him it was not that *I could not* do the call but that *I did not want to do that to myself* any longer. That I had value beyond this service and also that I would need to give up this job I loved if the alternative was giving up on myself. I certainly had privilege in the moment to know I could find other work, and yet, it was not a privilege I had conceived of using up to that point. I only knew to do what was expected of me. My resilience in that moment was giving my body what it was asking for instead of asking *of it to give yet more.*

Your resilience can look different every day because you are constantly shifting, transforming, and learning what your body needs and what you need to nurture it. And although you did not ask for or deserve any hardship, you can refuse to lose your humanity in how you rise to meet it. In fact, reclaiming yourself as a full and complex human may be the greatest resilience of all.

You may choose to answer with—

Rest: Yes, this includes physical rest, naps, pausing. It is also breath, laughter, self-love, scrolling less, taking in less information, and so much more. It is anything that puts you back in your body, where Justice lives. Resting in your body, to me, also means accepting its emotions, sensations, limitations, and triumphs, accepting what your body needs and lovingly giving it. Rest is saying no to additional requests that do not move your river of Joy. It is the antidote to the external noise and a triumphant choice to favor your inner awareness.

Take a Pause

With her Nap Ministry, Tricia Hersey has defiantly and beautifully redefined rest as a revolutionary movement. She has integrated deeply into her body a call to Justice by living and breathing what has been taken from her (and all of us) by white supremacy. Her work is inspiring and, in my opinion, the embodiment of resilience.

Anger: Your anger is your tuning in to what you feel and to what you resist. You can follow it for wisdom on how to move forward.

Grace: For yourself first of all. And then for others. For this world and all its complexities. Each time you offer grace, you create more space for your full human self to occupy.

Sadness: The ways you grieve and mourn loss, large and small, are reflections of your capacity to love. They are your bold will to engage with the world before you.

Gratitude: At times, for the pain itself, and at others, for your defiance to thrive through it. Gratitude, in the many forms we have discussed in this book, as a path to Justice in your body.

Take a Pause

Recall that gratitude is a way to also reclaim the past, especially if it was painful, as kindling for your present path. Gratitude for your ancestors will land you squarely in your body, defiant and resilient, all at the same time.

You can answer the call for resilience with any of these and so much more. The dictionary says resilience means you are *elastic* and *flexible*, coming back to your own normal after a stressor. But you rarely feel like *yourself* again after life is permanently changed by grief, oppression, or pain. Those broken wounds are, as Rumi writes, *where the light gets in*.

When you are fighting to stay human in an inhumane world, resilience feels crucial to reclaim. You can come back to *your new normal*, each time. You grow, learn, and evolve to be a new version of yourself that has incorporated all the pain, Joy, sadness, and laughter into a broken-open and expanded self. And the way you answer the call for resilience will change you as well.

What if you aren't supposed to *bounce back* after a challenge but instead *walk forward* toward your truth? What if your resilience is feeling your pain, the injustices, and *still*, as Maya Angelou says, *you rise*? And I do not think she meant you always feel good in your rising or that you make it through, but that you always know your value and worth to be bigger than the tragedy that tried to destroy it. And *still you rise*, no matter what, to meet the needs of your body each day. Your resilience is your own Chardi Kala.

Your rising is not one that negates the injustice in your life or this world. It acknowledges all that, all your challenging emotions, and still defiantly cries out that your Joy in this world is your proof that you can grow and thrive through the cracks of these larger systems and those of your heart. You do not survive to eventually rise. No, your rising is *how you survive.* And maybe, just maybe, somewhere, somehow, your rejoicing is lightening the souls of any of your ancestors who toiled and grieved and never knew that Joy was still theirs to have.

PRACTICE: TAKE A PAUSE AND CHECK IN

Literally take a pause. This practice is simple but not always easy to do. How do you check in with yourself, especially when life is hard, to know what your body needs? How do you listen with your full envelope? It is best done in ways that feel natural for you. You may want to meditate, you may want to write, move, pull tarot cards, draw, dance, swim, paint, anything that helps you pause and look within. Try to do it daily. It then becomes an act of self-love, to tend to your body. I take my pause in the early hours of the morning before the house is awake, through movement and breath. Find *your* body's best ways to ask for its most resilient action before the world asks it of you.

CHAPTER 20

In the Unknown

The COVID-19 pandemic was and remains, at the writing of this book, a landmark experience of uncertainty. Not nearly the first time any of us alone have felt unsure, but as a universal collective, the first in my lifetime that we are facing the same unknown *together.* My mentor, Debbie, gifted me an image that has stayed my steadfast companion through the unknown. I was contemplating an anxiety-provoking career transition and I explained I was learning to meet my fear anyway. I was feeling quite spiritually mature when I said it felt like I was being chased by an animal toward a cliff, but I saw myself still taking a big leap and feeling even, at times, exhilarated by it. Per her usual, Debbie found a lesson of higher truth and asked me to exchange my image for a gentler, more loving one.

What if, instead of that, you are standing at that cliff, and there is a wide, golden tightrope across the abyss? And then you walk out onto this luminous bridge. You are stable, safe, and held lovingly by the unknown beneath you.

This image required faith and love for that abyss and for myself as a capable, trusting being to cross it. The unknown could be my friend, a benefactor even, and hold me the entire time. When you practice Joy as a way of holding all that you feel, you cultivate that deeper faith in yourself. Not only that you are held but that you *deserve* to be held and comforted.

The science shows that when you face uncertainty, your brain perceives threat. You are a calculating, cognitive being who likes to know what lies around the next corner. And when you cannot predict or have been scarred by what awaited you before, you turn on your hypervigilant nervous system and highlight your limbic system where fear resides. And remember that your overaroused limbic system reduces the capacity of your frontal cortex to have clarity on how to turn that corner in the first place. This may explain why my initial image involved running, frightened, toward the cliff instead of the next one where I stood at it calmly and saw an alternate possibility. The possibilities for good and calm are reduced when your threatened nervous system takes over.

Uncertainty is not part of life, *it is life*. None of us ever knows what comes next, ever. Global pandemic or not. The more you can learn to not only live with but thrive through it, the more you will feel like you are stepping into life instead of away from it. And some of us, myself included, are more agitated than others in the midst of uncertainty. They sometimes call us *highly sensitive*. I take that not as a flaw but as a superpower. It means that I am in tune to my environment; my anxiety and fear are parts of my radar in this world. It doesn't mean I love feeling that way! But I can use them as signals from my body's radar, messages to listen to but not be consumed by. It means I know that I am not broken but instead whole in my humanity.

What if even in the most uncertain of times, you knew that amid your fear, worry, and anger there lay one certain truth? That

Joy is still yours to have. That you have the inner resources to cultivate a piece of that Joy, no matter how small, as a touchstone that this tide of uncertainty is a teacher for, but not a destroyer of, your Joy. That this uncertainty may make your heart tremble, but that same quiver also signifies that *the full potential of possibility* lives here. What if even when you do not know what lies in front of you, you deeply know instead *what lies within you*: a vast well of power and Justice that you give yourself, even when the world remains too shaky to offer it first?

I sometimes practice a meditation I call My Wise Council in uncertain moments. No surprise, Debbie first introduced me to a version of this. Recently, I offered it to one of the participants I am still working with from the Ukraine training. It was in the context of feeling a lack of community and love around her after having to leave her country for safety from the war. I met again with her last week, and she shared with me the beautiful image she received when doing this practice. No council of individuals appeared to her, instead she saw a lake and river that flow near her temporary home in Romania. She imagined herself floating in these waters, *calm, supported, and free*, she said. Nature was her council, her wide, golden sling in this uncertain and fearful time. You never know what piece of Justice your body will offer.

Take a Pause

Uncertainty and the unknown can be mirrors to your Joy practice, instead of something to dread; they can teach you how to stay open and deepen faith and trust, in yourself and life itself. When you expect the worst or cringe at what the next step will be, take a deep breath and exhale slowly. Activate that stillness within you and say to yourself in whatever language or wording works for you, *This fear is not all of who I am. I also have the capacity for faith and trust.* Until you believe it in your core. You can weave a wide, golden tightrope underneath as you pass through this.

In that vision of my Pashi Masi, she gave me my assignment, to use this life as my teacher so that I could look within and find my own Justice. I saw her again two years ago, in the same wise guide meditation, at the same creek in the woods. I was overjoyed to see her after more than a decade. Inside, my heart beat faster in anticipation that perhaps, she would give me my next life-altering instruction.

This time, I remained standing before her. I had no question, no words came out. I merely looked into her eyes, as real as the first time. The silence just as still. She cradled my chin and right cheek with one hand, smiled, and said, *You are doing it,* beti *(my child), you are doing it.* Shabash *(nice work).*

PRACTICE: YOUR WISE COUNCIL

This practice can be a touchstone in times of uncertainty. You can turn to it in any situation: financial stress, relationship troubles, career dissatisfaction, or even spiritual uncertainty in the face of loss or challenge. You can create a council of elders, wise sages, anyone who you feel has counsel for your next steps. And ask them questions.

1. Sit and attend to your breath to calm your nervous system. Close your eyes if able.
2. Breathe in and out three to five times, deeply, lengthening your exhale if possible.
3. Imagine a council of wise individuals sitting before you. They are wise and learned in the particular challenge you are facing. Maybe they are financially successful if you are having questions on money or they are people who have had success in healing from incredible loss. You do not need to know them personally. They can be people from your life or more famous ones you have not met yet.
4. Imagine them sitting across from you and that they are sending you love and acceptance.
5. Inhale their love and breathe out gratitude for this opportunity. Do this as many times as you need to really feel safe and settled in their company.
6. When you feel ready, ask them a question. What to do next, or best advice on your particular challenge. See what they offer. Listen with your whole envelope.
7. Stay here as long as you like or need. Take the messages with gratitude.
8. You can come back anytime and can have different councils for different issues. They can all be part of your wide, golden bridge through uncertainty.

CHAPTER 21

Your Joy Is Also Our Justice

It feels overwhelming to wrap up a book on such ineffable concepts as Joy and Justice, maybe because there is never an end point to either, only a calling for both to be fully expressed in as many ways as possible. And yet, I have a need to offer that although your own personal Justice is and always has been the purpose of this writing, I hope you sense that the inevitable outcome of you sustaining your personal revolution is that your path weaves into the world you inhabit. I did not expect or hold this to be true at first. In fact, I almost revolted against it. My Justice work in the world was often tiring, and not only could I not imagine how my spiritual seeking of Joy would at all intersect with such an exhausting effort, but the thought left me with guilt when others were suffering. Once I embarked seriously on the path to Joy, I understood that as a human right, the practice of Joy *is* Justice work in and of itself.

The more you love your sacred self, the more you know deeply that you deserve Joy in all its forms, the more the world will feel your power and radiance. What is good in the world will be made even better. But also, what is wrong with the world will have more of your clarity and action poured into it. Your revolution cannot help but be contagious; it's a law of quantum physics.

And trust me, this was not an outcome I was seeking. I was only preoccupied with my own spiritual journey to find Joy after traumatic grief. The more I reclaimed my birthright of Joy, the more I realized the freedom to seek Joy for Joy's sake alone. Not to be a better mother, physician, wife, friend, or sister. Not to be better in my work. Not for anyone or anything else. *But for the simple and ineffable reason that I am a sacred human being trying to live in a difficult world, and I deserve to have and feel Joy, no matter what.* And remember, the work of seeking Joy will be a piece of Justice to transform generations that have both walked before and those yet to come.

I was walking in my very hilly neighborhood and spotted a man with a young teenage woman in a wheelchair, her body contorted in a way that spoke of a condition severe enough for me to know she was likely unable to leave that chair independently. He was tilting her backward to safely and gently navigate the steep downhill, a maneuver I knew all too well. I was across the street heading in the opposite direction, uphill. And I had no ostensible reason to interact with them but felt compelled to do so.

I crossed the street to say hi and encourage him on this challenging walk. We shared only about five minutes of conversation, but in that time, he revealed how much his daughter loved being in the water and that the difficulty of the hills were worth the Joy of seeing her in the lake below. I shared my son also used a wheelchair, which noticeably eased the man's shoulders in a way that I knew meant he did not have to explain the layers of complexity this otherwise mundane walk with a child represented. We went on our ways, but before we did he looked me deeply in the eyes and thanked me for stopping and talking to them. And I did the same.

What you may see in this story is a short chat between strangers on a walk. But what passed between us was nothing short of a revolution. I, accessing my Joy as a regular practice, was able to linger in the awe of seeing father and daughter rolling down that hill as a sign of dedicated love. I was able to feel in my heart the simple beauty that when they finally reached the water, his daughter would feel freedom of movement in her body, floating in the warm summer sun. I was able to feel gratitude for that moment of connection between two parents who love fiercely yet also feel exhausted by the life they have been given. And who knows, he may have gone on to pass that moment of connection to another when he reached the lake.

In the same way that your pain is a bridge to feeling compassion for the pain of all beings, your Joy, too, is a bridge. When you feel it as a work of Justice, it is then an offering to the larger world. This life is hard and at times, downright treacherous. There is no doubt. But it is also full of opportunities for Joy. Not a cognitive experience of happiness, but the moment to moment, immediate sensation of Joy right here, right now in your body. Anytime you enter into even that smallest possible sliver, you access that deep river of knowing that you were meant to *rejoice* along with your suffering, that you always have been and always will be deserving of Joy. The more you sound that bell, the more you will say to the world that you are here, still standing, in all of your rage, power, sadness, and as well, your magnificent Joy. And that is the sound of sweet Justice.

Acknowledgments

The task of offering gratitude on a page feels daunting. If I were pressed to a few words, I would simply thank the ancestors who tended to and cultivated the soul I inhabit and the land I live on. The ancestors who gave us the wisdom, traditions, and practices that call us to see and know ourselves in the deepest of ways. The Justice warriors who fought for their Joy so that I can have the privilege to fight for mine. Any grace I have is, as Alice Walker says, *a measure of what has gone before.*

I could never express enough gratitude to those who have taught me about Justice and why it matters. To my patients and group participants, some of whom you met in this book, for trusting me with the privilege of witnessing your most vulnerable and inspiring moments and reminding me why fighting the inequities of the health-care system is as paramount as fighting disease. To my forever work family at Swedish Cherry Hill FMR, faculty and residents, past and present: you are light workers who practice medicine that matters. To Jim Gordon, the faculty, and staff at CMBM: our work together in the world has been one of my deepest teachers and fundamentally changed my life. To my fierce and inspiring Seattle community of South Asian sister activists who have created a Justice family of the very best kind, from the early days of Chaya and beyond—in particular, Manka Dhingra,

Rujuta Gaonkar, Charu Wahi, Uma Rao, Shelly Krishnamurthy, Manka Varghese, Aaliyah Gupta, and Pramila Jayapal.

For all the light workers in the book world who helped birth this dream. Who knew that a young Brown girl could dream about writing a book, and then one day, others would believe in her too? Bhu Srinivasan, for igniting me to believe that this book mattered. Linda Sivertsen, my book midwife, who shepherded my vision, and created a circle of writers (Kim Lowe, Shira Lilley, Jo Courtney, Marie Ruzicka) who held my dream dear. To my agent, Leslie Meredith, who fiercely believed in this book from day one. To the entire Hachette Go team, the dedicated elves you don't see—Mary Ann Naples, Michael Barrs, Sharon Kunz, Ashley Kiedrowski, Alison Dalafave, Iris Bass, Cisca Schreefel, and Terri Sirma. (You all have endless patience!) And with extra love, to my editor, Renee Sedliar. You are a magic maker. Not just your exquisite skill, but your advocacy, love, and capacity to see this book's power, all made you my steadfast touchstone. I felt so safe in your wise hands.

To other unique touchstones of Joy along the way. I am indebted to Debra Kaplan's wisdom and guidance, but, Debbie, I hope in some small way, it is even more palpable to you after you read this book. To my loving circles, for endless book support and those who did the extra work of holding my tender vulnerability of putting my deepest heart out into the world. Your energy is imprinted in this book with love—in particular: Ellen Vora, Drew Ramsey, Timara Freeman-Young, Ilene Ruhoy, Avanti Kumar-Singh, Michael Bays, Tara Clark, Maisha Davis, Adair Look, Jenny Phelps, Blanche and Nanette Olivar.

To my wider Seattle and global families, who hold our family in ways that allow us to hold it all. Too many to name, but the gifts are endless—from the far away calls and loving texts to the nearby market dinners, game nights and long walks; from the Halloween costumes and dance parties, to the delicious dosas, and all in between, the gratitude is beyond these words. You love, celebrate, and grieve with us, and show up. Every. Single. Time. And a special mention for a group who never gets recognition for their relentless work as Zubin's guardian angels in school and camps along the way. You have no idea how the way you held him also held Steve and me through so many rough times, but here is finally, my one chance to tell you. In particular, Mark Fraley, Andrew Chapman, Jordan Swanson, Glenn Brooks, Cheick Keita, Jean Nelson, Sandra Powell, Carol Aoki-Kramer, Mary Cohan, James Rees, Gregory Barnes, Blake Saunders, Natalie Gress, Jeremy Frye, Devon Lopes, Jose Luis Munoz and Sue Apkon. Community and love matter.

Gratitude is an inadequate word when it comes to my family, in particular, my parents, Surjit and Kaval Sethi, who have literally only lived and worked for the good of their children and grandchildren, persevered through so much, and continually pour endless love to us, no matter what. Your parenting is more like seva, which I won't even try to translate here because it wouldn't do you Justice.

My brothers and sisters-in-law—Robbie and Hansmeet Sethi, Reet Sidhu, and Sapna Mysoor— who are often my biggest cheerleaders and a soft place to land and laugh when I need, even about the horrible things. A special shout-out to Hansmeet and Sapna, for moving here and giving us family support we so desperately needed. Caring for a disabled child is not easy or simple, and having you here still brings me to as many tears as the first night you told me you were coming. To my beloved extended in-laws, both my Filipino and Desi circles (both of my sisters-in-law's families whom I love as my own): The way you all hold me dear is more life-giving than I can explain. And to my Mor-mor and Bestefar, who would have been so very proud.

To my babies who are no longer such—Sahaj, Zubin, and Neha—I get teary thinking of the intricate ways you have each taught me why Joy really matters. Through your challenges and triumphs, you are my soul's medicine. If I could let you know in any infinitesimal way how your love carves deep rivers through me, I would put it in a capsule for you to open anytime you need a reminder of your deep goodness. Thank you each for choosing me. May I be a good ancestor for you. Of course, to Nola, for your endless cuddles. And to Steve: There are no words, truly, for this beautiful, painful, vibrant life we have walked into together. For your laughter, tenderness, and endless ways you have poured into and nourished me through it all. You have never flinched once when it comes to my dreams, as if they were yours all the while. You will always be my *home*, where I go for refuge, to flourish, and to know that I am both loved and can love so deeply.

And lastly, only because I want you to really hear this— to you, the reader. If it weren't for you, for your belief that Joy is your birthright, that Justice is not only deeply needed in your body but in the world, this book would not have given birth. If it has touched any place in your heart, I am deeply grateful for that space. Our liberation is, and always has been, intricately woven together. May we all ring the bells of Justice for ourselves, and one another.

Notes

A Road Map

xxx **On my website.** Many exercises in the book are offered in guided audio format on my website: www.tanmeetsethimd.com.

xxxi **the heart and the gut have been described in mainstream medical literature.** J. A. Armour, *Neurocardiology: Anatomical and Functional Principles*, HeartMath Research Center, HeartMath Institute, Publication No. 03-011, 2003; M. Carabotti et al., "The Gut-Brain Axis: Interactions Between Enteric Microbiota, Central and Enteric Nervous Systems," *Annals of Gastroenterology* 28, no. 2 (April–June 2015): 203–209, PMID: 25830558, PMCID: PMC4367209.

Chapter 1: Does Joy Matter?

5 **Magic like less depression.** J. W. Pennebaker, "Writing About Emotional Experiences as a Therapeutic Process," *Psychological Science* 8 (1997): 162–166; R. Procaccia et al., "Benefits of Expressive Writing on Healthcare Workers' Psychological Adjustment During the COVID-19 Pandemic," *Frontiers in Psychology* 12 (February 25, 2021): 624176, http://doi.org:10.3389/fpsyg.2021.624176, PMID: 33716890, PMCID: PMC7947213; J. W. Pennebaker, J. K. Kiecolt-Glaser, and R. Glaser, "Disclosure of Traumas and Immune Function: Health Implications for Psychotherapy," *Journal of Consulting and Clinical Psychology* 56, no. 2 (1988): 239–245, https://doi.org/10.1037/0022-006X.56.2.239.

5 **chronic diseases, such as asthma or rheumatoid arthritis.** J. M. Smyth et al., "Effects of Writing About Stressful Experiences on Symptom Reduction in Patients with Asthma or Rheumatoid Arthritis: A Randomized Trial," *JAMA* 281, no. 14 (199914): 1304–1309.

6 **One of the most prolific.** James W. Pennebaker, "Expressive Writing in Psychological Science," *Perspectives in Psychological Science* 13, no. 2 (2018): 226–229.

7 **The science supports that you carve new pathways.** H. Parthasarathy, "You Can Teach an Old Owl New Tricks," *Nature*, September 2002, https://doi.org/10.1038/news020916-11.

7 **That sigh signals to your body.** G. J. Taylor, R. M. Bagby, and J. D. Parker, "Expressing Emotions Can Be Better for Your Health: The Alexithymia Construct. A Potential Paradigm for Psychosomatic Medicine," *Psychosomatics* 32, no. 2 (Spring 1991): 153–164, https://doi.org/10.1016/s0033-3182(91)72086-0, PMID: 2027937.

12 **When you reveal this deeper layer to yourself.** C. J. Wakslak and Y. Trope, "Cognitive Consequences of Affirming the Self: The Relationship Between Self-Affirmation and Object Construal," *Journal of Experimental Social Psychology* 45, no. 4 (2009): 927–932, https://doi.org/10.1016/j.jesp.2009.05.002.

12 **When you know this why, your brain comes back.** J. D. Creswell et al., "Affirmation of Personal Values Buffers Neuroendocrine and Psychological Stress Responses," *Psychological Science* 16, no. 11 (November 2005): 846–851, https://doi.org/10.1111/j.1467-9280.2005.01624.x, PMID: 16262767.

Chapter 2: You're Not Broken

16 **Resmaa Menakem refers to it as the *soul nerve*.** Resmaa Menakem, *My Grandmother's Hands: Racialized Trauma and the Pathway to Mending Our Hearts and Bodies* (Las Vegas: Central Recovery Press, 2017).

16 **you are also more likely to remember bad memories.** R. F. Baumeister et al., "Bad Is Stronger Than Good," *Review of General Psychology* 5, no. 4 (2001): 323–370, https://doi.org/10.1037/1089-2680.5.4.323.

16 **Stephen Porges, who developed the *polyvagal theory*.** Stephen Porges introduced the polyvagal theory in 1994 and has written numerous articles and books. Stephen W. Porges, *Polyvagal Theory: Neurophysiological Foundations of Emotions, Attachment, Communication, and Self-Regulation* (New York: W. W. Norton, 2011).

18 **you may feel a jittery anxiety or hypervigilance before any calm.** K. Kozlowska et al., "Fear and the Defense Cascade: Clinical Implications and Management," *Harvard Review of Psychiatry* 23, no. 4 (2015): 263–287, https://doi.org/10.1097/HRP.0000000000000065.

19 **a process called *neuroception*.** S. W. Porges, "Neuroception: A Subconscious System for Detecting Threat and Safety," *Zero to Three: Bulletin of the National Center for Clinical Infant Programs* 24, no. 5 (2004): 19–24; S. W. Porges, "The Polyvagal Theory: New Insights into Adaptive Reactions of the Autonomic Nervous System," *Cleveland Clinic Journal of Medicine* 76, suppl. 2 (2009): S86–S90, https://doi.org/10.3949/ccjm.76.s2.17.

19 ***interoceptive awareness*.** H. D. Critchley, "Neural Mechanisms of Autonomic, Affective, and Cognitive Integration," *Journal of Comparative Neurology* 493 (2005): 154–166.

19 **the science shows that when you perceive unfairness in life.** G. Novembre, M. Zanon, and G. Silani, "Empathy for Social Exclusion Involves the

Sensory-Discriminative Component of Pain: A Within-Subject fMRI Study," *Social Cognitive and Affective Neuroscience* 10, no. 2 (February 2015): 153–164, https://doi.org/10.1093/scan/nsu038, Epub February 21, 2014, PMID: 24563529, PMCID: PMC4321615.

19 **You can also feel a bodily threat from not feeling that you belong.** Claude M. Steele, "Thin Ice: 'Stereotype Threat' and Black College Students," *Atlantic Monthly*, August 1999, 44–47, 50–54; C. M. Steele and J. Aronson, "Stereotype Threat and the Intellectual Test Performance of African-Americans," *Journal of Personality and Social Psychology* 69 (1995): 797–811.

19 **Your body receives this pain of social exclusion.** M. D. Lieberman and N. I. Eisenberger, "The Dorsal Anterior Cingulate Cortex Is Selective for Pain: Results from Large-Scale Reverse Inference," *Proceedings of the National Academy of Sciences* 112, no. 49 (2015): 15250–15255; N. I. Eisenberger, M. D. Lieberman, and K. D. Williams, "Does Rejection Hurt? An fMRI Study of Social Exclusion," *Science* 302, no. 5643 (October 10, 2003): 290–292, https://doi.org/10.1126/science.1089134, PMID: 14551436.

20 **you may not feel as deserving of Joy.** C. M. Steele, "A Threat in the Air: How Stereotypes Shape the Intellectual Identities and Performance of Women and African-Americans," *American Psychologist* 52 (1997): 613–629.

21 **The anger and pain from feeling invisible can put you in that *fight-or-flight* state.** J. J. Gross and R. W. Levenson, "Hiding Feelings: The Acute Effects of Inhibiting Negative and Positive Emotion," *Journal of Abnormal Psychology* 1997, no. 1 (February 1997): 95–103, https://doi.org/10.1037//0021-843x.106.1.95, PMID: 9103721.

Chapter 3: The Present Moment Is Not Enough

30 **As I'm writing this book, a new study showed.** K. N. Fitzgerald et al., "Potential Reversal of Epigenetic Age Using a Diet and Lifestyle Intervention: A Pilot Randomized Clinical Trial," *Aging* (Albany, NY) 13, no. 7 (April 12, 2021): 9419–9432, https://doi.org/10.18632/aging.202913, Epub April 12, 2021.

30 **So, if you're a Black woman.** B. J. Goosby and C. Heidbrink, "Transgenerational Consequences of Racial Discrimination for African American Health," *Sociology Compass* 7, no. 8 (2013): 630–643.

31 **Rachel Yehuda has shown.** R. Yehuda and L. M. Bierer, "Transgenerational Transmission of Cortisol and PTSD Risk," *Progress in Brain Research* 167 (2008): 121–135, https://doi.org/10.1016/S0079-6123(07)67009-5, PMID: 18037011.

31 **Some argued that maybe.** R. Yehuda, A. Lehrner, and L. M. Bierer, "The Public Reception of Putative Epigenetic Mechanisms in the Transgenerational Effects of Trauma," *Environmental Epigenetics* 4, no. 2 (July 17, 2018): dvy018, https://doi.org/10.1093/eep/dvy018, PMID: 30038801, PMCID: PMC6051458;

A. Lehrner et al., "Intergenerational Effects of Maternal Holocaust Exposure on *FKBP5* Methylation," *American Journal of Psychiatry* 177, no. 8 (August 1, 2020): 744–753, https://doi.org/10.1176/appi.ajp.2019.19060618.

31 **in 2013, a study showed that mice.** B. Dias and K. Ressler, "Parental Olfactory Experience Influences Behavior and Neural Structure in Subsequent Generations," *Nature Neuroscience* 17 (2014): 89–96, https://doi.org/10.1038/nn.3594.

32 **So, yes, Kayla can do breathwork.** S. Venditti et al., "Molecules of Silence: Effects of Meditation on Gene Expression and Epigenetics," *Frontiers in Psychology* 2020 (August 11, 2020): 1767, https://doi.org/10.3389/fpsyg.2020.01767.

33 **manage her stress in a way that folds or unfolds these proteins.** R. Lambrot et al., "Low Paternal Dietary Folate Alters the Mouse Sperm Epigenome and Is Associated with Negative Pregnancy Outcomes," *Nature Communications* 4, no. 2889 (December 2013); U. Sharma et al., "Biogenesis and Function of tRNA Fragments During Sperm Maturation and Fertilization in Mammals," *Science* 351, no. 6271 (January 22, 2016): 391–396, https://doi.org/10.1126/science.aad6780; Q. Chen et al., "Sperm tsRNAs Contribute to Intergenerational Inheritance of an Acquired Metabolic Disorder," *Science* 351, no. 6271 (January 22, 2015): 397–400, https://doi.org/10.1126.

37 **But the studies clearly show.** A. Kalambouka et al., "The Impact of Placing Pupils with Special Educational Needs in Mainstream Schools on the Achievement of Their Peers," *Educational Research* 49, no. 4 (2007): 365–382.

37 **children have less prejudice.** Gordon W. Allport, *The Nature of Prejudice* (New York: Basic Books, 1979).

Chapter 4: Your Body Knows

50 **Jim Gordon, MD, conducts a small mind body medicine skills group.** Dr. Gordon is the founder of the Center for Mind Body Medicine, www.cmbm.org, where I am on faculty and have learned my small group facilitation work with groups experiencing trauma. In the book, the subsequent mind body medicine trainings I reference were done as faculty with CMBM. Find more information on its website in how to participate in its global-wide trainings.

Chapter 5: Rewrite the System

62 **Science is catching up to what the ancient sages have known.** A. Berkovich-Ohana et al., "Repetitive Speech Elicits Widespread Deactivation in the Human Cortex: The 'Mantra' Effect?" *Brain Behavior* 5, no. 7 (July 2015): e00346, https://doi.org/10.1002/brb3.346, Epub May 4, 2015, PMID: 26221571, PMCID: PMC4511287.

62 **Especially if you hum or chant a mantra.** B. G. Kalyani et al., "Neurohemodynamic Correlates of 'OM' Chanting: A Pilot Functional Magnetic Resonance Imaging Study," *International Journal of Yoga* 4, no. 1 (2011): 3–6, https://doi.org/10.4103/0973-6131.78171; J. Gao et al., "The Neurophysiological Correlates of Religious Chanting," *Scientific Reports* 9, no. 4262 (2019).

65 **The best neuroplasticity.** B. A. Linkenhoker and E. I. Knudsen, "Incremental Training Increases the Plasticity of the Auditory Space Map in Adult Barn Owls," *Nature* 419 (2002): 293–296.

66 **When you imagine what you want in the future.** C. N. Cascio et al. "Self-affirmation Activates Brain Systems Associated with Self-Related Processing and Reward and Is Reinforced by Future Orientation," *Social Cognitive and Affective Neuroscience* 11, no. 4 (2016): 621–629, https://doi.org/10.1093/scan/nsv136; L. B. Pham and S. E. Taylor, "From Thought to Action: Effects of Process-Versus Outcome-Based Mental Simulations on Performance," *Personality and Social Psychology Bulletin* 25, no. 2 (1999): 250–260, https://doi.org/10.1177/0146167299025002010.

66 **you can strengthen muscles.** B. C. Clark et al., "The Power of the Mind: The Cortex as a Critical Determinant of Muscle Strength/Weakness," *Journal of Neurophysiology* 112, no. 12 (December 15, 2014): 3219–3226, https://doi.org/10.1152/jn.00386.2014, Epub October 1, 2014, PMID: 25274345, PMCID: PMC4269707.

66 **have more success if they practice their skill.** S. Arora et al., "Mental Practice Enhances Surgical Technical Skills: A Randomized Controlled Study," *Annals of Surgery* 253, no. 2 (February 2011): 265–270, https://doi.org/10.1097/SLA.0b013e318207a789, PMID: 21245669; A. Pascual-Leone et al., "Modulation of Muscle Responses Evoked by Transcranial Magnetic Stimulation During the Acquisition of New Fine Motor Skills," *Journal of Neurophysiology* 74, no. 3 (September 1995): 1037–1045, https://doi.org/10.1152/jn.1995.74.3.1037, PMID: 7500130.

Chapter 6: Ask, Don't Tell

75 **Amy Cuddy.** Amy Cuddy, "Your Body Language May Shape Who You Are," TED Talk, June 2012, https://www.ted.com; her book is *Presence: Bringing Your Boldest Self to Your Biggest Challenges* (New York: Little, Brown and Company, 2015); D. R. Carney, A. J. Cuddy, and A. J. Yap, "Power Posing: Brief Nonverbal Displays Affect Neuroendocrine Levels and Risk Tolerance," *Psychological Science* 21, no. 10 (October 2010): 1363–1368, https://doi.org/10.1177/0956797610383437, Epub September 20, 2010, PMID: 20855902.

75 **People simply feel.** S. L. and T. F. P. Arnette, "The Effects of Posture on Self-Perceived Leadership," *International Journal of Business and Social Science* 3, no.

4 (2012); A. H. Bailey et al., "Could a Woman Be Superman? Gender and the Embodiment of Power Postures," *Comprehensive Results in Social Psychology* 2 (2016): 6–27.

75 **there is evidence that individuals with power and status.** Robert Sommer, *Personal Space: The Behavioral Basis of Design* (Englewood Cliffs, NJ: Prentice Hall, 1969).

76 **When oppression and chronic microaggressions are studied in communities.** Rae Johnson et al., "The Embodied Experience of Microaggressions: Implications for Clinical Practice," *Journal of Multicultural Counseling and Development* 46, no. 3 (July 2018): 156–170, https://doi.org/10.1002/jmcd.12099.

76 **In fact, these chronic bodily aggressions.** Babette Rothschild, *The Body Remembers: The Psychophysiology of Trauma and Trauma Treatment* (New York: W. W. Norton, 2000).

77 **Maya Angelou's life-changing words.** Maya Angelou, "Still I Rise," in *And Still I Rise: A Book of Poems* (New York: Random House, 1978).

77 **I heard Amy Cuddy speak on a podcast.** *Bouncing Forward with Amy Purdy*, Anchor, https://anchor.fm/amy-purdy1/episodes/Amy-Cuddy-Living-Inspired-Through-Uninspiring-Times-and-The-Importance-Of-Supporting-One-Another-e1bvdgc/a-a74jr60.

80 **When you suppress your emotions.** P. R. Goldin et al., "The Neural Bases of Emotion Regulation: Reappraisal and Suppression of Negative Emotion," *Biological Psychiatry* 63 (2008): 577–586.

80 **when your limbic system is aroused.** J. Gross, "Emotion Regulation: Affective, Cognitive, and Social Consequences," *Psychophysiology* 39 (2002): 281–291.

81 **there is a technique that neuroscience has shown.** J. J. Gross and O. P. John, "Individual Differences in Two Emotion Regulation Processes: Implications for Affect, Relationships, and Well-Being," *Journal of Personality and Social Psychology* 85, no. 2 (2003): 348–362; M. D. Lieberman et al., "Putting Feelings into Words: Affect Labeling Disrupts Amygdala Activity in Response to Affective Stimuli," *Psychological Science* 18, no. 5 (2007): 421–428.

82 **Matthew Lieberman, a neuroscientist at UCLA.** J. B. Torre and M. D. Lieberman, "Putting Feelings into Words: Affect Labeling as Implicit Emotion Regulation," *Emotion Review* 10, no. 2 (2018): 116–124.

86 **psychiatrist Viktor Frankl's.** Viktor E. Frankl, *Man's Search for Meaning: An Introduction to Logotherapy*, 4th ed. (Boston: Beacon Press, 1992).

Chapter 7: Don't Just Accept Everything

94 **In my TEDx Talk.** Tanmeet Sethi, "Two Words That Can Change Your Life," TedxRainier, November 2015; you can watch it at www.tanmeetsethimd.com.

Chapter 8: Your Love Matters

102 **It supports that vagal pathway of safety.** S. W. Porges, "Vagal Pathways: Portals to Compassion," in *The Oxford Handbook of Compassion Science*, ed. E. M. Seppälä et al. (New York: Oxford University Press, 2017), 189–202.

102 **If you want a teen to change a habit.** O. Longe et al., "Having a Word with Yourself: Neural Correlates of Self-Criticism and Self-Reassurance," *Neuroimage* 49, no. 2 (January 15, 2010): 1849–1856, https://doi.org/10.1016/j.neuroimage.2009.09.019, Epub September 18, 2009, PMID: 19770047.

102 **Harsh words signal your midbrain centers to be fearful.** P. Gilbert, "Evolutionary Approaches to Psychopathology: The Role of Natural Defences," *Australian & New Zealand Journal of Psychiatry* 35, no. 1 (2001): 17–27, https://doi.org/10.1046/j.1440-1614.2001.00856.x.

103 **Researchers show through sophisticated brain imaging.** Longe et al., "Having a Word with Yourself."

103 **In fact, when you extend compassion to yourself.** O. Ayduk and E. Kross, "From a Distance: Implications of Spontaneous Self-Distancing for Adaptive Self-Reflection," *Journal of Personality and Social Psychology* 98, no. 5 (May 2010): 809–829, https://doi.org/10.1037/a0019205, PMID: 20438226, PMCID: PMC2881638; E. Seppala, T. Rossomando, and J. Doty, "Social Connection and Compassion: Important Predictors of Health and Well-Being," *Social Research* 80, no. 2 (2013): 411–430; H. Chapin et al., "Compassion Meditation Training for People Living with Chronic Pain and Their Significant Others: A Pilot Study and Mixed-Methods Analysis," *Journal of Compassionate Healthcare* 1, no. 4 (2014); https://doi.org/10.1186/s40639-014-0004-x, Epub October 27, 2014; H. Jazaieri et al., "A Randomized Controlled Trial of Compassion Cultivation Training: Effects on Mindfulness, Affect, and Emotion Regulation," *Motivation and Emotion* (2013).

108 **Kristin Neff, one of the pioneering researchers.** "One of the Three Elements of Self-Compassion," Self-Compassion.org, https://self-compassion.org/the-three-elements-of-self-compassion-2/.

110 **The science of touch supports this invitation.** K. Uvnäs-Moberg, "Oxytocin May Mediate the Benefits of Positive Social Interaction and Emotions," *Psychoneuroendocrinology* 23, no. 8 (November 1998): 819–835, https://doi.org/10.1016/s0306-4530(98)00056-0, PMID: 9924739; M. Eckstein et al., "Calming Effects of Touch in Human, Animal, and Robotic Interaction—Scientific State-of-the-Art and Technical Advances," *Frontiers in Psychiatry* 4 (November 4, 2020): 11:555058, https://doi.org/10.3389/fpsyt.2020.555058.

110 **Functional MRI (fMRI) studies.** J. A. Coan, H. S. Schaefer, and R. J. Davidson, "Lending a Hand: Social Regulation of the Neural Response to

Threat," *Psychological Science* 17, no. 12 (2006): 1032–1039, https://doi.org/10.1111/j.1467-9280.2006.01832.x.

Chapter 9: Your Body Is Your Home; Settle In

115 **Being in your whole envelope, an *embodied* approach.** F. Fiori, N. David, and S. M. Aglioti, "Processing of Proprioceptive and Vestibular Body Signals and Self-Transcendence in Ashtanga Yoga Practitioners," *Frontiers in Human Neuroscience* 8 (September 18, 2014): 734, https://doi.org/10.3389/fnhum.2014.00734, PMID: 25278866, PMCID: PMC4166896.

116 **When you hug someone.** K. Uvnäs-Moberg, "Oxytocin May Mediate the Benefits of Positive Social Interaction and Emotions," *Psychoneuroendocrinology* 23, no. 8 (November 1998): 819–835, https://doi.org/10.1016/s0306-4530(98)00056-0, PMID: 9924739.

117 **Even the touch of warm temperature.** L. E. Williams and I. A. Bargh, "Experiencing Physical Warmth Promotes Interpersonal Warmth," *Science* 322, no. 5901 (October 24, 2008): 606–607, https://doi.org/10.1126/science.1162548, PMID: 18948544, PMCID, PMC2737341.

117 **Researchers have studied yoga practitioners.** Fiori, David, and Aglioti, "Processing of Proprioceptive and Vestibular Body Signals"; N. A. Farb, Z. V. Segal, and A. K. Anderson, "Mindfulness Meditation Training Alters Cortical Representations of Interoceptive Attention," *Social Cognitive and Affective Neuroscience* 8, no. 1 (2014): 15–26, https://doi.org/10.1093/scan/nss066.

118 **As Etty Hillesum, who died in a Nazi concentration camp.** Etty Hillesum and Arnold Pomerans, *An Interrupted Life: The Diaries of Etty Hillesum 1941–1943* (New York: Pantheon Books, 1983).

119 **When you breathe deeply, you activate.** A. Zaccaro et al., "How Breath-Control Can Change Your Life: A Systematic Review on Psycho-Physiological Correlates of Slow Breathing," *Frontiers in Human Neuroscience* 12 (September 7, 2018): 353, https://doi.org/10.3389/fnhum.2018.00353, PMID: 30245619, PMCID: PMC6137615.

119 **When meditators bring attention to their breath.** K. A. Garrison et al., "Meditation Leads to Reduced Default Mode Network Activity Beyond an Active Task," *Cognitive, Affective & Behavioral Neuroscience* 15, no. 3 (September 2015): 712–720, https://doi:.org/10.3758/s13415-015-0358-3, PMID: 25904238, PMCID: PMC4529365.

120 **Most acute emotions will pass through the body in a minute or two.** Jill Bolte Taylor, *My Stroke of Insight: A Brain Scientist's Personal Journey* (New York: Viking, 2008).

120 **use your breath to *ride it out*.** S. Bowen and A. Marlatt, "Surfing the Urge: Brief Mindfulness-Based Intervention for College Student Smokers," *Psychology of*

Addictive Behaviors 23, no. 4 (2009): 666–671, https://doi.org/10.1037/a0017127; B. D. Ostafin and G. A. Marlatt, "Surfing the Urge: Experiential Acceptance Moderates the Relation Between Automatic Alcohol Motivation and Hazardous Drinking," *Journal of Social and Clinical Psychology* 27, no. 4 (2008): 404–418, https://doi.org/10.1521/jscp.2008.27.4.404.

124 **The evidence that trauma takes up residence.** Bessel van der Kolk, *The Body Keeps the Score: Brain, Mind, and Body in the Healing of Trauma* (New York: Viking, 2014).

125 **It occurs microscopically as well.** R. K. Naviaux, "Metabolic Features of the Cell Danger Response," *Mitochondrion* 16 (May 2014): 7–17, https://doi.org/10.1016/j.mito.2013.08.006, Epub August 24, 2013, PMID: 23981537.

129 **It is also a powerful drug in the brain.** M. N. Hill et al., "Endogenous Cannabinoid Signaling Is Required for Voluntary Exercise-Induced Enhancement of Progenitor Cell Proliferation in the Hippocampus," *Hippocampus* 20, no. 4 (April 2010): 513–523, https://doi.org/10.1002/hipo.20647, PMID: 19489006, PMCID: PMC2847038.

129 **Movement also increases a sophisticated neurochemical in the brain.** S. Bathina and U. N. Das, "Brain-Derived Neurotrophic Factor and Its Clinical Implications," *Archives of Medical Science* 11, no. 6 (December 10, 2015): 1164–1178, https://doi.org/10.5114/aoms.2015.56342, Epub December 11, 2015, PMID: 26788077, PMCID: PMC4697050.

130 **holistic psychiatrist Ellen Vora.** Ellen Vora, *The Anatomy of Anxiety: Understanding and Overcoming the Body's Fear Response* (New York: Harper Wave, 2022).

131 **Music does literally move you.** C. L. Gordon, P. R. Cobb, and R. Balasubramaniam, "Recruitment of the Motor System During Music Listening: An ALE Meta-analysis of fMRI Data," *PLoS One* 13, no. 11 (November 19, 2018): e0207213, https://doi.org/10.1371/journal.pone.0207213, PMID: 30452442, PMCID: PMC6242316.

131 **It stimulates dopamine and endorphins.** V. Salimpoor et al., "Anatomically Distinct Dopamine Release During Anticipation and Experience of Peak Emotion to Music," *Nature Neuroscience* 14 (2011): 257–262, https://doi.org/10.1038/nn.2726.

131 ***Hope molecules.*** C. Phillips and A. Salehi, "A Special Regenerative Rehabilitation and Genomics Letter: Is There a 'Hope' Molecule?" *Physical Therapy* 96, no. 4 (April 2016): 581–583, https://doi.org/10.2522/ptj.2016.96.4.581, PMID: 27037293.

132 **Practice: Shaking and Dancing Meditation.** I first learned this version I am teaching in my work with the Center for Mind Body Medicine, but as with all ancient expressive meditations, no one owns these practices and we have all borrowed them with humility from our ancestors.

133 "**Brokedown Palace.**" Lyrics: Robert Hunter, music: Jerry Garcia, 1970.

134 **this kind of movement puts us *in sync*.** B. Tarr, J. Launay, and R. I. Dunbar, "Silent Disco: Dancing in Synchrony Leads to Elevated Pain Thresholds and Social Closeness," *Evolution and Human Behavior* 37, no. 5 (2016): 343–349, https://doi.org/10.1016/j.evolhumbehav.2016.02.004; B. Tarr, J. Launay, and R. I. Dunbar, "Music and Social Bonding: 'Self-Other' Merging and Neurohormonal Mechanisms," *Frontiers in Psychology* 5 (September 30, 2014): 1096, https://doi.org/10.3389/fpsyg.2014.01096.

135 **Even just one ninety-minute walk.** G. N. Bratman et al., "Nature Experience Reduces Rumination and Subgenual Prefrontal Cortex Activation," *Proceedings of the National Academy of Sciences* (USA) 112, no. 28 (July 14, 2015): 8567–8572, https://doi.org/10.1073/pnas.1510459112, Epub June 29, 2015, PMID: 26124129, PMCID: PMC4507237.

135 **And a walk among trees.** M. Antonelli et al., "Effects of Forest Bathing (Shinrin-yoku) on Levels of Cortisol as a Stress Biomarker: A Systematic Review and Meta-analysis," *International Journal of Biometeorology* 63, no. 8 (August 2019): 1117–1134.

135 **my family and I joined forty-five-plus others.** For more information on accessible caminos, look up the incredible work of I'll Push You at https://www.illpushyou.com.

139 **The neuroscience supports that even small rituals.** A. W. Brooks et al., "Don't Stop Believing: Rituals Improve Performance by Decreasing Anxiety," *Organizational Behavior and Human Decision Processes* 137 (2016): 71–85.

139 **You can assign more meaning to a ritual.** M. I. Norton and F. Gino, "Rituals Alleviate Grieving for Loved Ones, Lovers, and Lotteries," *Journal of Experimental Psychology: General* 143 (2014): 266.

Chapter 10: Hope for Yourself

145 **I remember his words.** Zak Cheney-Rice, "Bryan Stevenson on His 'Not Entirely Rational' Quest for Justice," *New York Magazine*, July 2019, https://nymag.com/intelligencer/2019/06/bryan-stevensons-not-entirely-rational-quest-for-justice.html.

149 **Hope as well has been shown to improve well-being, heart health.** C. C. Schiavon et al., "Optimism and Hope in Chronic Disease: A Systematic Review," *Frontiers in Psychology* 7 (January 4, 2017): 2022, https://doi.org/10.3389/fpsyg.2016.02022; R. J. Reichard et al., "Having the Will and Finding the Way: A Review and Meta-analysis of Hope at Work," *Journal of Positive Psychology* 8, no. 4 (2013): 292–304, https://doi.org/10.1080/17439760.2013.800903.

149 **One study parsed out the two concepts.** F. B. Bryant and J. A. Cvengros, "Distinguishing Hope and Optimism: Two Sides of a Coin, or Two Separate Coins?" *Journal of Social and Clinical Psychology* 23, no. 2 (2004): 273–302, https://doi.org/10.1521/jscp.23.2.273.31018.

150 **It has been linked to happiness.** Schiavon et al., "Optimism and Hope in Chronic Disease."

150 **and even a strong predictor of mortality.** M. F. Scheier and C. S. Carver, "Adapting to Cancer: The Importance of Hope and Purpose," in *Psychosocial Interventions for Cancer*, ed. Andrew Baum and Barbara L. Andersen (Washington, DC: American Psychological Association, 2001), 15–36, https://doi.org/10.1037/10402-002.

150 **in one study of three hundred–plus.** M. F. Scheier et al., "Optimism and Rehospitalization After Coronary Artery Bypass Graft Surgery," *Archives of Internal Medicine* 159, no. 8 (1999): 829–835, https://doi.org/10.1001/archinte.159.8.829.

150 **Hope, to me, is the foundation of the placebo effect.** A. Girac, A. Aamir, and P. Zis, "The Neurobiology Under the Placebo Effect," *Drugs Today* (Barcelona) 55, no. 7 (July 2019): 469–476, https://doi.org/10.1358/dot.2019.55.7.3010575, PMID: 31347615; I. Požgain, Z. Požgain, and D. Degmečić, "Placebo and Nocebo Effect: A Mini-Review, *Psychiatria Danubina* 26, no. 2 (June 2014): 100–107, PMID: 24909245.

Chapter 11: Gratitude Doesn't Solve Everything

156 **And it doesn't count to be grateful.** R. A. Emmons and M. E. McCullough, "Counting Blessings Versus Burdens: An Experimental Investigation of Gratitude and Subjective Well-Being in Daily Life," *Journal of Personality and Social Psychology* 84, no. 2 (February 2003): 377–389, https://doi.org/10.1037//0022-3514.84.2.377, PMID: 12585811.

156 **Studies show that people who do something as simple.** Robert A. Emmons and Michael E. McCullough, *The Psychology of Gratitude* (New York: Oxford University Press, 2004).

157 **There are a couple of tweaks that seem to uplevel this practice.** B. H. O'Connell et al., "Feeling Thanks and Saying Thanks: A Randomized Controlled Trial Examining If and How Socially Oriented Gratitude Journals Work," *Journal of Clinical Psychology* 73, no. 10 (October 2017): 1280–1300; N. M. Lambert et al., "Expressing Gratitude to a Partner Leads to More Relationship Maintenance Behavior," *Emotion* 11 (2011): 52–60.

157 **The science suggests that the more you express gratitude.** L. I. Hazlett et al., "Exploring Neural Mechanisms of the Health Benefits of Gratitude in Women: A Randomized Controlled Trial," *Brain, Behavior, and Immunity* 95

(July 2021): 444–453, https://doi.org/10.1016/j.bbi.2021.04.019, Epub April 28, 2021, PMID: 33932527; E. Perreau-Linck et al., "In Vivo Measurements of Brain Trapping of C-labelled Alpha-Methyl-L-tryptophan During Acute Changes in Mood States," *Journal of Psychiatry & Neuroscience* 32, no. 6 (November 2007): 430–434, PMID: 18043767, PMCID: PMC2077345; R. Zahn et al., "The Neural Basis of Human Social Values: Evidence from Functional MRI," *Cerebral Cortex* 19, no. 2 (February 2009): 276–283, https://doi.org/10.1093/cercor/bhn080, Epub May 22, 2008, PMID: 18502730, PMCID: PMC2733324.

158 **It directly decreases your heart rate.** S. Kyeong et al., "Effects of Gratitude Meditation on Neural Network Functional Connectivity and Brain-Heart Coupling," *Scientific Reports* 7, no. 1 (July 11, 2017): 5058, https://doi.org/10.1038/s41598-017-05520-9, PMID: 28698643, PMCID: PMC5506019.

158 **people with heart failure do better.** P. J. Mills et al., "The Role of Gratitude in Spiritual Well-Being in Asymptomatic Heart Failure Patients," *Spirituality in Clinical Practice* (Washington, DC) 2, no. 1 (2015): 5–17, https://doi.org/10.1037/scp0000050; R. S. Redwine et al., "Pilot Randomized Study of a Gratitude Journaling Intervention on Heart Rate Variability and Inflammatory Biomarkers in Patients with Stage B Heart Failure," *Psychosomatic Medicine* 78, no. 6 (2016): 667–676, https://doi.org/10.1097/PSY.0000000000000316.

160 **you also produce oxytocin.** S. B. Algoe and B. M. Way, "Evidence for a Role of the Oxytocin System, Indexed by Genetic Variation in CD38, in the Social Bonding Effects of Expressed Gratitude," *Social Cognitive and Affective Neuroscience* 9, no. 12 (2014): 1855–1861, https://doi.org/10.1093/scan/nst182.

160 **And when you rewrite your experiences of gratitude in detail.** L. A. King and K. N. Miner, writing about the perceived benefits of traumatic events: "Implications for Physical Health," *Personality and Social Psychology Bulletin* 26 (2000): 220–230; L. S. Redwine et al., "Pilot Randomized Study of a Gratitude Journaling Intervention."

160 **if you can write about something you're grateful for twenty-one days in a row.** Y. J. Wong et al., "Does Gratitude Writing Improve the Mental Health of Psychotherapy Clients? Evidence from a Randomized Controlled Trial," *Psychotherapy Research* 28, no. 2 (March 2018): 192–202, https://doi.org/10.1080/10503307.2016.1169332, Epub May 3, 2016, PMID: 27139595.

160 **This practice can amplify the effects of therapy alone.** Wong et al., "Does Gratitude Writing Improve the Mental Health of Psychotherapy Clients?"

161 **Studies also show that writing a gratitude letter.** P. Kini et al., "The Effects of Gratitude Expression on Neural Activity," *Neuroimage* 128 (March 2016): 1–10, https://doi.org/10.1016/j.neuroimage.2015.12.040, Epub December 30, 2015, PMID: 26746580; M. Henning et al., "A Potential Role for mu-Opioids in Mediating the Positive Effects of Gratitude," *Frontiers in Psychology* 8,

no. 868 (2017), https://doi.org/10.3389/fpsyg.2017.00868; Martin E. P. Seligman, *Flourish: A Visionary New Understanding of Happiness and Well-Being* (New York: Atria, 2013).

161 **psychologist Martin Seligman.** Seligman, *Flourish*.

162 **Practice: The Gratitude Visit.** Adapted from Seligman, *Flourish*.

162 **The studies show that even when you listen.** G. R. Fox, "Neural Correlates of Gratitude," *Frontiers in Psychology* 6, no. 1491 (2015), https://doi.org/10.3389/fpsyg.2015.01491.

165 **Studies map out its effects in the brain.** M. Henning et al., "A Potential Role for mu-Opioids."

165 **Gratitude can help you *assign your own new meaning*.** The way you reframe a traumatic story: K. N. Ochsner et al., "Rethinking Feelings: An fMRI Study of the Cognitive Regulation of Emotion," *Journal of Cognitive Neuroscience* 14, no. 8 (November 15, 2002): 1215–1229, https://doi.org/10.1162/089892902760807212, PMID: 12495527; P. Watkins et al., "Taking Care of Business? Grateful Processing of Unpleasant Memories," *Journal of Positive Psychology* 3, no. 2 (2008): 87–99, https://doi.org/10.1080/17439760701760567.

166 **After the World Trade Center attacks on 9/11.** B. L. Fredrickson et al., "What Good Are Positive Emotions in Crises? A Prospective Study of Resilience and Emotions Following the Terrorist Attacks on the United States on September 11th, 2001," *Journal of Personality and Social Psychology* 84, no. 2 (2003): 365–376, https://doi.org/10.1037//0022-3514.84.2.365.

166 **This kind of *making meaning out of suffering*.** D. P. McAdams, "The Psychology of Life Stories," *Review of General Psychology* 5 (2001): 100–122; D. P. McAdams et al., "When Bad Things Turn Good and Good Things Turn Bad: Sequences of Redemption and Contamination in Life Narrative and Their Relation to Psychosocial Adaptation in Midlife Adults and Students," *Personality and Social Psychology Bulletin* 27 (2001): 474–485.

167 **In one small study, gratitude practice.** P. Kini et al. "The Effects of Gratitude Expression on Neural Activity," *Neuroimage* 128 (March 2016): 1–10, http: doi.org/10.1016/j.neuroimage.2015.12.040, Epub December 30, 2015, PMID: 26746580.

167 **Practice: Gratitude Reappraisal.** Jeremy Adam Smith et al., *The Gratitude Project: How the Science of Thankfulness Can Rewire Our Brains for Resilience, Optimism, and the Greater Good* (Oakland, CA: New Harbinger Publications, 2020).

Chapter 12: It's Not Forgiveness, It's Grace

176 **Chronic, unrelenting anger.** P. Schwenkmezger and P. Hank, "Anger Expression and Blood Pressure," in *Stress and Emotion: Anxiety, Anger, and Curiosity*,

ed. Charles D. Spielberger and Irwin G. Sarason (Washington, DC: Taylor & Francis, 1996), vol. 16, 241–259; S. R. Wenneberg et al., "Anger Expression Correlates with Platelet Aggregation," *Behavioral Medicine* 22 (1997): 174–177; C. E. Thoresen, F. Luskin, and A. H. A. Harris, "Science and Forgiveness Interventions: Reflections and Recommendations," in *Dimensions of Forgiveness*, ed. Everett L. Worthington Jr. (Philadelphia: Templeton Foundation Press, 1998), 163–190.

176 **Your stress hormones go down.** Frederic Luskin, *Forgive for Good: A Proven Prescription for Health and Happiness* (San Francisco: Harper, 2002).

178 **Researchers describe a practice called psychological distancing.** G. F. Giesbrecht, U. Müller, and M. Miller, "Psychological Distancing in the Development of Executive Function and Emotion Regulation," in *Self and Social Regulation: Social Interaction and the Development of Social Understanding and Executive Functions*, ed. Bryan W. Sokol et al. (New York: Oxford University Press, 2010), 337–357; I. E. Sigel, "The Psychological Distancing Model: A Study of the Socialization of Cognition," *Culture & Psychology* 8, no. 2 (2002): 189–214.

178 **Studies show it helps you diffuse the emotional charge.** J. S. Moser et al., "Third-Person Self-Talk Facilitates Emotion Regulation Without Engaging Cognitive Control: Converging Evidence from ERP and fMRI," *Scientific Reports* 7, no. 4519 (2017), https://doi.org/10.1038/s41598-017-04047-3.

178 **If you see a situation as a threat, you go into stress mode.** A. L. Alter et al., "Rising to the Threat: Reducing Stereotype Threat by Reframing the Threat as a Challenge," *Journal of Experimental Social Psychology* 46, no. 1 (2010): 166–171, https://doi.org/10.1016/j.jesp.2009.09.014; J. P. Jamieson, W. B. Mendes, and M. K. Nock, "Improving Acute Stress Responses: The Power of Reappraisal," *Current Directions in Psychological Science* 22, no. 1 (2013): 51–56, https://doi.org/10.1177/0963721412461500; J. J. Blascovich et al., "The Biopsychosocial Model of Arousal Regulation," *Advances in Experimental Social Psychology* 28 (1996): 1–51.

179 **One study showed that even thinking.** C. vanOyen Witvliet, T. E. Ludwig, and K. L. Vander Laan, "Granting Forgiveness or Harboring Grudges: Implications for Emotion, Physiology, and Health," *Psychological Science* 12, no. 2 (March 2001): 117–123, https://doi.org/10.1111/1467-9280.00320, PMID: 11340919.

179 **One is to create space.** Y. Trope, N. Liberman, and C. Wakslak, "Construal Levels and Psychological Distance: Effects on Representation, Prediction, Evaluation, and Behavior," *Journal of Consumer Psychology* 17, no. 2 (2007): 83–95.

180 **Or you can create space with time.** Y. Trope and N. Liberman, "Temporal Construal," *Psychological Review* 110, no. 3 (2003): 403.

181 **When we *reappraise* the stories of the wrongs or tragedy.** P. C. Watkins et al., "Taking Care of Business? Grateful Processing of Unpleasant Memories," *Journal of Positive Psychology* 3, no. 2 (2008): 87–99, https://doi.org/10.1080/17439760701760567.

Chapter 14: In Awe

190 **The science shows that moments of awe.** J. E. Stellar et al., "Self-Transcendent Emotions and Their Social Functions: Compassion, Gratitude, and Awe Bind Us to Others Through Prosociality," *Emotion Review* 9, no. 3 (2017): 200–207, https://doi.org/10.1177/1754073916684557; E. J. Horberg, C. Oveisand, and D. Keltner, "Emotions as Moral Amplifiers: An Appraisal Tendency Approach to the Influences of Distinct Emotions upon Moral Judgment," *Emotion Review* 3 (2011): 1–8; D. Keltner and J. Haidt, "Approaching Awe, a Moral, Spiritual, and Aesthetic Emotion," *Cognition and Emotion* 17 (2003): 297–314, https://doi.org/10.1080/02699930302297.

190 **An interesting and so artfully simple study with Berkeley students.** P. K. Piff et al., "Awe, the Small Self, and Prosocial Behavior," *Journal of Personality and Social Psychology* 108, no. 6 (2015): 883–899, https://doi.org/10.1037/pspi0000018.

191 **Dacher Keltner.** Keltner and Haidt, "Approaching Awe."

191 **Melanie Rudd.** M. Rudd, K. D. Vohs, and J. Aaker, "Awe Expands People's Perception of Time, Alters Decision Making, and Enhances Well-Being," *Psychological Science* 23, no. 10 (October 1, 2012): 1130–1136, https://doi.org/10.1177/0956797612438731, Epub August 10, 2012, PMID: 22886132.

191 **Jennifer Stellar.** J. E. Stellar, "Awe Helps Us Remember Why It Is Important to Forget the Self," *Annals of the NY Academy of Sciences* 1501, no. 1 (October 2021): 81–84, https://doi.org/10.1111/nyas.14577, Epub February 5, 2021, PMID: 33547655.

191 **the literature describes how moments of awe lower inflammation.** J. E. Stellar et al., "Positive Affect and Markers of Inflammation: Discrete Positive Emotions Predict Lower Levels of Inflammatory Cytokines," *Emotion* 15, no. 2 (January 19, 2015): 129–133, advance online publication (2012), http://doi.org/10.1037/emo0000033.

192 **Science has now found.** D. B. Yaden et al., "The Varieties of Self-Transcendent Experience," *Review of General Psychology* 21, no. 2 (2017): 143–160, https://doi.org/10.1037/gpr0000102.

192 **when I read about the *overview effect*.** D. B. Yaden et al., "The Overview Effect: Awe and Self-Transcendent Experience in Space Flight," *Psychology of*

Consciousness: Theory, Research, and Practice 3, no. 1 (2016): 1–11, https://doi.org/10.1037/cns0000086.

192 **that astronauts have likened that now iconic view.** D. B. Yaden et al., "The Overview Effect: Awe and Self-Transcendent Experience," in Frank White, *Space Flight; The Overview Effect: Space Exploration and Human Evolution* (New York: Houghton and Mifflin, 1987); *Bulletin of Science, Technology & Society* 8, no. 4 1988): 453–454.

193 **German astronaut Sigmund Jähn.** Yaden et al., "The Overview Effect."

193 **Awe also takes you out of your ruminating mind.** M. van Elk et al., "The Neural Correlates of the Awe Experience: Reduced Default Mode Network Activity During Feelings of Awe," *Human Brain Mapping* 40, no. 12 (August 15, 2019): 3561–3574, https://doi.org/10.1002/hbm.24616, Epub May 7, 2019, PMID: 31062899, PMCID: PMC6766853.

193 **A study of older individuals, between the ages of sixty and ninety.** V. E. Sturm et al., "Big Smile, Small Self: Awe Walks Promote Prosocial Positive Emotions in Older Adults," *Emotion* 22, no. 5 (August 2022): 1044–1058, https://doi.org/10.1037/emo0000876, Epub September 21, 2020, PMID: 32955293, PMCID: PMC8034841.

194 **And you are changed because of it.** R. Janoff-Bulman, "Posttraumatic Growth: Three Explanatory Models," *Psychological Inquiry* 15 (2004): 30–34.

194 **Practice: Awe Walk/Roll/Watch.** V. E. Sturm et al., "Big Smile, Small Self."

Chapter 15: In Beauty

196 **Science quantifies beauty by a wonderful term, an *aesthetic chill*.** R. R. McCrae, "Aesthetic Chills as a Universal Marker of Openness to Experience," *Motivation and Emotion* 31, no. 1 (2007): 5–11, https://doi.org/10.1007/s11031-007-9053-1.

196 **When you appreciate beauty.** T. Ishizu and S. Zeki, "Toward a Brain-Based Theory of Beauty," *PLoS One* 6, no. 7 (2011): e21852, https://doi.org/10.1371/journal.pone.0021852.

197 **those higher on the openness scale.** C. R. Jonassaint et al., "Facets of Openness Predict Mortality in Patients with Cardiac Disease," *Psychosomatic Medicine* 69, no. 4 (May 2007): 319–322, https://doi.org/10.1097/PSY.0b013e318052e27d, Epub May 17, 2007, PMID: 17510289.

197 **brain scans show that these individuals.** P. G. Williams et al., "Individual Differences in Aesthetic Engagement Are Reflected in Resting-State fMRI Connectivity: Implications for Stress Resilience," *Neuroimage* 179 (October 1, 2018): 156–165, https://doi.org/10.1016/j.neuroimage.2018.06.042, Epub June 17, 2018, PMID: 29908310, PMCID: PMC6410354.

Chapter 16: In Faith

199 **In 1662, *Atocha*, a Spanish ship.** Philip J. Hilts, "Seeds Sprout After 365 Years in Sea," *Washington Post*, June 23, 1987, https://www.washingtonpost.com/archive/politics/1987/06/23/seeds-sprout-after-365-years-in-sea/36860d64-fec2-4c7c-b9e1-6e078cb0bc8f/.

Chapter 18: In Your Purpose

206 **studies show that people with a sense of purpose sleep better.** A. Alimujiang et al., "Association Between Life Purpose and Mortality Among US Adults Older Than 50 Years," *JAMA Network Open* 2, no. 5 (May 3, 2019): e194270, https://doi.org/10.1001/jamanetworkopen.2019.4270, PMID: 31125099, PMCID: PMC6632139; R. Cohen, C. Bavishi, and A. Rozanski, "Purpose in Life and Its Relationship to All-Cause Mortality and Cardiovascular Events: A Meta-analysis," *Psychosomatic Medicine* 78, no. 2 (February–March 2016): 122–133, https://doi.org/10.1097/PSY.0000000000000274, PMID: 26630073.

206 **One of the most common psychological scales.** Ryff Scales of Psychological Well-Being.

207 **Researchers describe a sense of purpose.** Anthony Burrow, principal investigator, "Intervening on Purpose and Meaning in Adolescence," Bronfenbrenner Center for Translational Research, Pilot Study Program—Cornell University; R. Sumner, A. L. Burrow, and P. L. Hill, "The Development of Purpose in Life Among Adolescents Who Experience Marginalization: Potential Opportunities and Obstacles," *American Psychologist* 73, no. 6 (September 2018): 740–752, https://doi.org/10.1037/amp0000249, PMID: 30188163.

207 **And those who face the most adversity.** C. D. Ryff, C. L. Keyes, and D. L. Hughes, "Status Inequalities, Perceived Discrimination, and Eudaimonic Well-Being: Do the Challenges of Minority Life Hone Purpose and Growth?" *Journal of Health and Social Behavior* 44, no. 3 (September 2003): 275–291, PMID: 14582308.

Chapter 19: In Resilience

209 **A study in first-year resident physicians.** K. K. Ridout et al., "Physician-Training Stress and Accelerated Cellular Aging," *Biological Psychiatry* 86, no. 9 (November 1, 2019): 725–730, https://doi.org/10.1016/j.biopsych.2019.04.030, Epub May 9, 2019, PMID: 31230727, PMCID: PMC6788968.

210 **Science has shown that they get shorter with stressors.** E. S. Epel et al., "Accelerated Telomere Shortening in Response to Life Stress," *Proceedings of the National Academy of Sciences* (USA) 101, no. 49 (December 7, 2004): 17312-5,

https://doi.org/10.1073/pnas.0407162101, Epub December 1, 2004, PMID: 15574496, PMCID: PMC534658; K. K. Ridout et al., "Early Life Adversity and Telomere Length: A Meta-analysis," *Molecular Psychiatry* 23, no. 4 (April 2018): 858–871, https://doi.org/10.1038/mp.2017.26, Epub March 21, 2017, PMID: 28322278, PMCID: PMC5608639.

212 **With her Nap Ministry.** Theologian and author Tricia Hersey: https://the napministry.wordpress.com @thenapministry on Instagram.

Chapter 20: In the Unknown

216 **The science shows that when you face uncertainty.** M. Hsu et al., "Neural Systems Responding to Degrees of Uncertainty in Human Decision-Making," *Science* 310, no. 5754 (December 9, 2005): 1680–1683, https://doi.org/10.1126/science.1115327, PMID: 16339445.

Index